Communication Skills for Professional Nurses

Communication Skills for Professional Nurses

MICHAEL P. PAGANO

SANDRA L. RAGAN

with Deborah Booton, R.N.

SAGE PUBLICATIONS
International Educational and Professional Publisher
Newbury Park London New Delhi

For information address:

SAGE Publications, Inc.
2455 Teller Road
Newbury Park, California 91320

SAGE Publications Ltd.
6 Bonhill Street
London EC2A 4PU
United Kingdom

SAGE Publications India Pvt. Ltd.
M-32 Market
Greater Kailash I
New Delhi 110 048 India

Printed in the United States of America

Library of Congress Cataloging-in-Publication Data

Pagano, Michael P.
    Communication skills for professional nurses / Michael P. Pagano, Sandra L. Ragan, with Deborah Booton.
        p.   cm.
    Includes bibliographical references and index.
    ISBN 0-8039-4556-6 (cl).—ISBN 0-8039-4557-4 (pb)
    1. Communication in nursing.   2. Interpersonal communication.
3. Nursing—Social aspects.   I. Ragan, Sandra L.   II. Booton, Deborah.   III. Title.
    [DNLM: 1. Communication—nurses' instruction.
2. Interprofessional Relations—nurses' instruction.   3. Nurses—
Patient Relations.   WY 87 P131c]
    RT23.P34   1992
    610.73'06'99—dc20
    DNLM/DLC   92-7628

92   93   94   95   10   9   8   7   6   5   4   3   2   1

Sage Production Editor: Diane S. Foster

Contents

Epigraph

"Nursing is the diagnosis and treatment of *human responses* [italics added] to actual or potential health problems."

(AMERICAN NURSES' ASSOCIATION, 1980, p. 9)

Foreword

I am pleased to have participated in the development and creation of this unique communication textbook for nurses. As both an Assistant Professor in a College of Nursing and a practicing Family Nurse Practitioner, I am excited about this text. I am convinced that it will be a welcome addition to the corpus of information available to nursing students, both undergraduate and graduate, nursing faculty, practicing nurses, and nursing administrators. I find this book extremely useful because it contributes to both a theoretical understanding of the communication process and to enhancing the reader's communication skills through the use of practical examples that relate to a wide variety of everyday nursing experiences.

As we all know, verbal communication begins at birth and nonverbal communication starts in utero. These most basic communication traits form the foundation for the skills needed for all human interaction. Throughout our lives we utilize verbal and nonverbal as well as written communication skills, to inform and persuade others. As nurses, we are totally dependent upon our ability to communicate in order to fulfill the countless responsibilities of our profession. I can think of no other skill that is as universal to all aspects of nursing practice and so intrinsically necessary to the accomplishment of the art and science of nursing. This essential tool of our trade, however, is often relegated to only a few paragraphs in most nursing textbooks, a smattering of lecture hours, and an occasional "process recording." It is frequently assumed that by virtue of life experiences and college preparation nursing students have a sufficient understanding of the communication process to have developed the communication skills needed to effectively interact with patients, peers, and others. In addition, continued expansion of the nursing curricula often relegates "communication courses" to a cursory or nonexistent level. This minimal attention to enhancing nurses' communication skills and understanding of the communication process often persists in the work place, where ACLS training is frequently viewed as more vital than enhancing one's communication skills. Yet, we must realize that in order to be effective professionals at every level of patient, peer, or physician interaction, we need to be effective communicators.

I believe this text provides information and practical applications that can enhance nurses' communication skills and improve their understanding of the communication process. This book can be used by undergraduate nursing students, graduate students, nursing faculty, practicing nursing professionals, and nursing administrators to assist them in becoming more effective speakers, listeners, and writers. This text accomplishes these goals by providing a theoretical understanding of the communication process and by offering countless examples and exercises to enhance the reader's communication skills in order to develop more effective communication between nurses and patients, peers, physicians, and others.

DEBORAH BOOTON, PH.D., R.N., R.N.C, F.N.P.
Assistant Professor
University of Oklahoma College of Nursing

Preface

The purpose of this text is to help you evaluate and improve your understanding of the communication process as well as your communication skills. This book is unique in several ways. First, it is intended to be used by all levels of professional nurses—from the classroom to the boardroom, at the bedside, and when authoring a medical record. Second, this volume is distinctive because it uses scenarios from actual practice settings as the basis for an interactive relationship between the reader and the text. Finally, this book is atypical because it is dedicated solely to communication behaviors and skills and covers all three types of communication—verbal, nonverbal, and written.

The authors bring to this text diverse medical and academic backgrounds. One of the authors has worked in medicine for more than a quarter of a century and developed a great appreciation for the difficult tasks of communicating a variety of information to disparate audiences in a wide array of formats. Both authors have taught, researched, and written about the need for effective communication. In addition, the nursing consultant for this text is both a member of a nursing school faculty and a Nurse Practitioner.

The onerous nature of professional nursing, especially in the last decade of the twentieth century, demands that nurses be competent communicators at countless levels. As you know, nurses are expected to be informative, persuasive, and compassionate speakers and writers as well as highly perceptive listeners and observers.

It is no longer possible for a nurse to work at a patient's bedside and communicate with only a patient and a physician.

Because of technological advances, societal changes, and government intervention, modern nursing is a complex and evolving profession that demands coherent and competent communicators to assure patients the best possible health care and to prevent malpractice litigation. With the introduction of Quality Assessment and the requirements of Diagnosis Related Grouping (DRG), nursing professionals are expected to assess, comfort, document, and treat patients with a wide variety of illnesses and conditions. Some of these duties are administrative in nature, but nonetheless critical to the goals and objectives of contemporary health care. Nurses today are required to communicate with a vast array of audiences—patients, patients' families, physicians, colleagues, supervisors, other members of the health care team, and hospital administrators— in order to accomplish their eclectic tasks.

This textbook is intended to aid you in communicating with these diverse audiences by illustrating how effective verbal, nonverbal, and written communication skills can help you to demonstrate your professional competency and credibility.

MICHAEL P. PAGANO, PH.D., P.A.
SANDRA L. RAGAN, PH.D.

1

Communication Behaviors

Example #1

It's 10 minutes before the end of Carol O'Hara's evening shift when the patient in room 575 pushes his call light. Ms. O'Hara enters the patient's room and notices that the man is crying. She goes to the side of his bed, turns off the call light, and then speaks to the patient, who is scheduled for a breast biopsy in the morning.

> *Nurse O'Hara*: "What did you need, Mr. Swenson?"
>
> *Mr. Swenson*: "I was wondering if you thought it was too late to call my doctor? I have a couple of questions about my surgery and I thought maybe she could answer them over the phone." The 40-year-old man spoke softly, but never raised his eyes off the sheets in front of him.
>
> *Nurse O'Hara*: "Well, it's pretty late. Dr. Lamaze isn't on call tonight, so why don't you get some sleep. I'm sure she'll be able to answer your questions when she comes by in the morning."

Carol tucked the pillow under the man's head, flipped off the light switch, and left the room. When she returned to the nurses' station, Carol considered making a note about the patient's questions, but it was late and the next shift was ready to count narcotics, so she hurried to the med room and forgot about Mr. Swenson's concerns.

This example, which we will return to later in the chapter, is not atypical of the many communication settings that nurses face on a daily basis. The purpose of this text is to help you use more effective verbal, nonverbal, and written communication when interacting and communicating health care information. In addition, we will focus on the complexities of communication competency, the role of persuasion in compliance-gaining strategies, methods for establishing credibility, as well as defining the transactional nature of communication.

Watzlawick, Bavelas, and Jackson (1967) believe that human beings "cannot not communicate" (p. 49). With that in mind, and, being cognizant of Berlo's (1960) belief that "all communication behavior has as its purpose the eliciting of a specific response," (p. 12) we can assess the ways in which communication behaviors accomplish or fail to achieve an intended response.

AUDIENCE

A major goal of effective communication is interpreting what messages are being communicated by others (i.e., peers, patients, families, physicians, etc.) and responding in an appropriate and informative manner. For health care professionals, especially nurses, the variety of audiences that must be observed, assessed, and responded to makes effective communication difficult, but not impossible.

One of the first assessments for an effective communicator is a determination of the intended audience for his or her communication. An audience in a health care setting may consist of patients, peers, physicians, other members of the health care team, patients' families, student nurses, supervisory personnel, administrators, or even lawyers. The level of education among these various audiences may range, at the extremes, from illiteracy to a doctoral degree. Therefore, an audience's ability to comprehend and respond appropriately to a nurse's message must be carefully considered by the nurse-speaker or nurse-writer.

For example, as a nurse, you should not explain a surgical procedure in the same manner to everyone who is about to undergo the same type of operation. The vocabulary (language choices) and syntax (the way words are put together to achieve a certain meaning) required to discuss an upcoming tonsillectomy with a 7-year-old patient should be different for the youngster than for his or her parents. Furthermore, the same procedure would, in all likelihood, have to be discussed differently still with a 32-year-old lawyer who was also having a tonsillectomy. Yet, many health care professionals memorize a speech that they deliver to all patients about an upcoming surgery, regardless of the patient's age, level of education, or cultural background.

In the space that follows please write a brief description of a tonsillectomy for a 7-year-old preop patient. Then rewrite that description for the child's parents, whom you believe to have a 12th-grade education. Finally, write a third paragraph describing the same operation for a lawyer who is scheduled for surgery the following day.

PERSUASION

As you discovered when you wrote the three descriptions, your language choices must be vastly different for the three audiences. A nurse who is explaining a tonsillectomy to a 7-year-old needs to inform the child about the events that will take place and assure the child that she or he will have fewer sore throats after the surgery. In addition, the nurse is trying to persuade the child that there will not be much pain, not too many needles, and lots of ice cream afterwards. The nurse wants to be informative but, at the same time, minimize the pain and maximize the postoperative benefits. The need for persuasion is just as strong in the nurse's discussion of the upcoming operation with the lawyer, but with this patient the nurse wants to persuade him or her that the staff, the physician, and the hospital are competent and credible and that the operation will be done expeditiously, correctly, and with a minimum of discomfort.

Both audiences need to be persuaded, but the communication behaviors, language choices, and nonverbal actions are vastly different for these two examples and demonstrate the dilemma faced by all nursing professionals.

Scholars have discussed the need for persuasion in communication since the time of Aristotle's *The Rhetoric* (1960). However, numerous writers since Aristotle, including Cicero (1949) and Kenneth Burke (1969a, 1969b), have also proclaimed the importance for speakers and writers to be persuasive in their interactions and writing. These authors focus on the importance of persuading an audience by demonstrating a speaker's competency and credibility. Prelli (1989) states, "scientific discourse is accepted or rejected on grounds of its reasonableness—given the issue at stake, the knowledge conditions of the scientific community, and the perceived expertise of the makers of the claims" (p. 7). It is the speaker's expertise that must be clearly demonstrated in both her or his verbal and nonverbal behaviors if an audience is to be persuaded.

Today, health care professionals are expected to demonstrate their competency through the care they provide to patients, the compassion they demonstrate, and the sound reasoning they communicate. A nurse's ability to persuade an audience that she or he is credible, competent, and compassionate ultimately affects a patient's opinion of both the nurse and the institution. More important, persuading an audience is critical to quality patient care. (In order to aid a patient's recovery, you need his or her assistance. It's difficult to treat an infected wound if the patient doesn't trust you enough to allow you to touch or handle the injured extremity. Persuading the patient that you are a competent, highly trained professional is an effective way to gain the patient's cooperation and compliance.) In addition, your ability to demonstrate through effective communication that you are a competent and credible nursing professional will help you to avoid the hassles of malpractice litigation. (Patients generally don't think about malpractice if they trust the person who is administering to their needs. All too frequently it's patients who feel that they are being depersonalized and dehumanized by care givers who respond with legal action.) Think about how you feel when you are ill. If your health care provider is curt and noninformative, and if you don't respond to the treatment, are you more likely to blame that provider or a provider who is compassionate, caring, and informative? If you are like most of us, you are willing to trust a person who persuades you through his or her communication that he or she is concerned about your health and competent to provide whatever health care services you need. Conversely, a provider who is unwilling to listen to your complaints or demonstrate any concern about your illness or your lack of response to treatment comes across as an uncaring, inhumane individual. As you probably know, people generally treat others as they feel they are being treated. If you, as a nurse, persuade someone that you are concerned, they will trust you. If you communicate your disinterest and lack of concern, the patient will be unconcerned about how his or her legal action might affect you.

As a health care professional who is constantly communicating with patients, patients' families, medical staff, peers, and others, you are expected to be astute in your ability to use verbal, nonverbal, and written communication to inform and persuade audiences. However, if you do not feel competent in these areas, you may be creating unnecessary problems for your patients and yourself.

COMMUNICATION COMPETENCY

One way to evaluate your ability to communicate is to assess your verbal communication competency. That is, are you able to use language choices and syntax that are appropriate for the audience you are addressing? Can you interpret an audience's understanding of your message and correct any misunderstandings? Are you able to use persuasion to assist you in communicating your information?

Your communication skills should provide you the ability to be a competent listener. For example, ask yourself whether you give an audience a chance to ask questions, or whether you are in such a hurry to deliver your message that you avoid an audience's responses? Do you use your powers of observation to assess an audience's nonverbal responses, as well as heeding their verbal cues? Can you evaluate the meaning of an audience's nonverbal behaviors: glance (facial expressions), timing (responses), kinesics (body movements), proxemics (distance between communicators), and haptics (touching behaviors)?

Finally, are you able to discern what your writing communicates to others? Do you read your written communication as a reader or as the document's author? When you author documents, are you trying to communicate specific information or are you merely trying to fill up the space on a page?

This text is dedicated to assisting you in becoming more aware and competent in each of these aspects of communication. It is our goal to help you discover how to assess and improve your verbal, nonverbal, and written competencies with a wide variety of audiences. Communication requires at least two individuals, but effective communication results from the interactants' willingness to use their communication competencies to ensure a successful exchange of information.

Now, let's go back to Example #1, the scenario that opened this chapter. In order to improve her communication competency, what are some of the verbal, nonverbal, and written behaviors that Nurse O'Hara might have changed? Please use the space below to briefly rewrite the segments of the encounter that you feel could have communicated more effectively to the patient. In addition, describe the aspects of the interaction that you feel are important to document for current and future users of the medical record.

Some of the areas you might have changed include: Ms. O'Hara demonstrating her concern for the patient's anxiety and/or sadness by asking about his tears, standing closer to his bed (proxemics), touching the patient's shoulder or hand (haptics), and using eye contact. She then would have nonverbally communicated her willingness to listen and respond to the patient's concerns. More than likely, the patient was anxious about his upcoming surgery, perhaps out of fear caused by a lack of knowledge about the procedure, the anesthesia risk, his postoperative recovery, the pain, or the possibility that his breast lump is a rare male breast cancer. The problem with the original example is that the nurse never attempted to discover and allay the patient's fears by asking him about his anxiety, discussing the procedure, or determining the patient's preparation for it. His anxiety was clearly demonstrated in his verbal and nonverbal communication, yet Ms. O'Hara never addresses these messages. In addition, the nurse fails to document the patient's concern and anxiety in the chart. This type of information could prove valuable to the patient's other nurses, the anesthesiologist or anesthetist, and the surgeon. All of these members of the health care team might be able to allay some of the patient's anxiety if they are aware of it. Without clear communication from one member of the team to another, however, this important patient information will remain unknown.

In the unforeseen event that something should go wrong in surgery or a complication occur following the procedure, an anxious preop patient is more likely to feel that the staff was incompetent and thereby responsible for a postop complication. Conversely, a patient who believes the staff is competent, compassionate, and concerned about his or her well-being, as demonstrated by their willingness to listen and exchange information, will be less likely to use them as scapegoats. The following chapters are intended to assist you in communicating with patients, families, and other members of the health care team. It is our desire to make your interactions and written communication more effective, and therefore more rewarding for you and those with whom you are communicating.

2

Fundamentals of Interpersonal Communication

The example in Chapter 1 illustrates some of the fundamentals of interpersonal communication. As that brief scenario demonstrates, the practice of nursing extensively involves the practice of communicating interpersonally. In fact, several widely accepted theoretical approaches to nursing include interpersonal communication as a key aspect of the nursing profession. Three of these approaches follow:

1. King's (1981) model views nursing as "a process of human interactions between nurse and client whereby each perceives the other and the situation; and through communication, they set goals, explore means, and agree on means to achieve goals" (p. 144).

2. Orlando (1961) writes of nursing as assisting patients in meeting their needs "through a process of deliberative interaction in which the nurse recognizes the verbal and nonverbal behavior indicative of unmet needs, validates those needs with the patient, and acts to meet the patient's needs" (p. 29).

3. Peplau (1952) sees nursing as "a significant, therapeutic, interpersonal process . . . an educative instrument, a maturing force, that aims to promote forward movement of [the] personality" (p. 16).

In all of these definitions and in most other theoretical approaches to nursing, interpersonal communication plays a pivotal role, so much so that one could forcefully argue that effective nursing relies on effective face-to-face communication.

THE TRANSACTIONAL NATURE OF INTERPERSONAL COMMUNICATION

How do you define interpersonal communication, and what are its components? Communication researchers, unfortunately, have not yet arrived at a common definition for communication, let alone for the slippery phenomenon of interpersonal communication. For the purposes of this text, however, we will adopt a widely held notion of interpersonal communication known as transactional theory. This theory posits that interpersonal communication is dyadic (consisting of two individuals), face-to-face communication in which each person emits cues—both verbal and nonverbal—and each assigns meaning to her or his own and the other's cues (Wilmot, 1987).

The notion of dyadic or two-party communication is the most generalized conception of interpersonal communication; however, few would argue that interpersonal communication does not take place as well in groups of three or more. Certainly the dyad is the locus for much of the communication in our daily lives that we would deem personal and is perhaps the only locus for intimate communication. In our professional lives as well, and in nursing, in particular, the dyad functions as the basic unit for communicating, whether it be nurse-patient, nurse-physician, nurse-family member, etc. Must interpersonal communication necessarily be face-to-face interaction? One could definitely argue that phone conversations can be interpersonal communication; again, however, we more commonly think of interpersonal communication as occurring in the actual presence of another.

Wilmot (1987) points to several important features of interpersonal communication:

1. It is transactional. This means that both participants influence and are influenced by the other. Their behaviors affect each other in the past, present, and future. The participants are involved in a communication process whereby meaning is jointly negotiated; one is not just passively receiving meaning from the other.

2. Each participant simultaneously encodes and decodes communication cues. That is, both people are continually emitting verbal and nonverbal messages and are continually trying to decipher the other's messages. Communication doesn't occur in a stop-start fashion where one party speaks and the other listens or one encodes and the other decodes. Think about how we actually talk and listen to each other. The two communicators are playing the roles of both speaker and listener, encoder and decoder, sender and receiver at the same time. This transactional view of communication counters the previously held approaches that envisioned communication from a linear, sender-receiver model. Perhaps you were taught in high school or college courses that communication is simply the process of transmitting information from one person to another. Seen this way, it makes sense to talk of these individuals as mere senders and receivers. Because we know that communication is an ongoing process wherein both participants are simultaneously sending and receiving, the unidirectional sender-receiver model is inadequate in explaining how the complex communication process functions.

3. In interpersonal communication, any action by one communicator can be seen as cause or effect by the other communicator, contingent on his or her point of view. In other words, because communication is a circular process rather than a linear one, it is difficult to argue in any objective sense that a particular communicative act is either a cause or an effect. Yet we hear people continually attributing their own communication behavior to another's prior behavior. For example, you might overhear a colleague, Nancy, say, "Every time I talk to Jan, I get so angry. She always says something that makes me mad." Nancy is expressing her belief that her anger is caused by Jan's behavior, but we must wonder what Jan might say about Nancy's assessment. Probably, Jan would regard her own communicative acts as a reaction to a prior behavior by Nancy. In other words, Jan believes that her actions represent the *effects* of Nancy's behavior and are not the *cause* of Nancy's anger.

Some communicators delight in playing the game of "you started it." For effective communication it is important to realize that such a game doesn't have winners because you are only arguing from your point of view. The better strategy is to focus on the situation or on the problem instead of viewing your own behavior as either caused by or in reaction to someone else's as if you didn't have a choice! For example, instead of trying to pin the blame for a mistake on someone, it is a much better strategy to try and determine what happened and how to correct the mistake. Blaming behaviors accomplish very little and usually serve no productive purpose. So when Nurse Tunes and Nurse Wyatt discover that Ms. Hayward's 1800 hours dressing change hasn't been done by 2115 hours, they can either blame each other, confront a third nurse, or they can get the patient's dressing changed and then try to determine what steps can be taken to prevent such an oversight from happening again. By taking care of the patient and trying to correct the cause of the problem, they avoid ineffective blaming behaviors and use effective communication to improve their delivery of quality care.

Why is it important for you, as a nursing professional, to see the communication process as a transactional one? Primarily because the Transactional Model more accurately describes communication between two parties than the Sender-Receiver approach. Further, the Transactional Model emphasizes the vital importance of mutual influence between the two communicators. Again, both affect the other's behavior, and both engage in a process of negotiating or determining the meaning of messages. You can influence your patient's willingness to comply with his or her self-care, for example, but the patient is still free to refuse your attempts at influence, and, in so doing, the patient may persuade you to change your strategies for eliciting her or his compliance.

The Transactional Model of communication also reminds us that the listening and interpreting functions of communication are of paramount importance to effective, accurate communication. Many communicators are convinced that if they speak effectively, use appropriate nonverbal cues, and if they are compassionate, persuasive, clear, and knowledgeable, their messages will always be accurately decoded. Of course this is not the case, because we are continually confronted by misunderstanding and a lack of cooperation, in both our personal and professional lives. We may be able to perfect our speaking and encoding skills, but this does not assure us that the people with whom we communicate will really hear what we are saying. Because accurate and effective communication relies as heavily on the other communicator as it does on us, we must take into account differences in the other (e.g., personal experience, culture, education, religion, etc.) as well as "noise" in the communication channels that might promote confusion and inaccurate decoding. Ineffective communication is often caused by our arrogance in believing that the other person sees the world through our lenses!

PERCEPTION OF THE OTHER

Because effective communication relies on our ability to accurately perceive the other person, a few words are in order about human perception. First of all, person perception is a complex phenomenon as no doubt you are already aware. Perceiving a surgical instrument is not so complex, simply because the act of perceiving is one-way; the instrument has no interest in perceiving you. Person perception involves a more convoluted set of relationships. You perceive someone; she or he perceives you; and the mutual act of perception affects both your perceptions. This is what Wilmot (1987) refers to as the transactional nature of interpersonal perception. It means that how we perceive an individual is a function not only of our own characteristics and biases, but also of the characteristics and biases of the other person. A person who claims to perceive others objectively is either ignorant or arrogant or both!

To further complicate matters, the way a person perceives us influences how we perceive them and vice versa. Perhaps this sounds like a hopeless conundrum, but the important thing to remember is that perception, like interpersonal communication, is a process wherein both parties influence each other. If you perceive a patient as being rude and noncompliant, your response to him or her may influence the patient, in turn, to perceive you as bossy and demanding. This perception will result in patient behavior that will "prove" your theory that she or he is rude and noncompliant! This perceptual circularity only leads to inaccuracy and misunderstanding.

How do we perceive people accurately? We first recognize that perception is subjective. We become aware of our prejudices and biases and guard against making judgments that confirm these. We remain open to the possibility that a person may disconfirm the stereotypes we have always associated with someone with her or his medical history, socioeconomic class, culture, religion, or family background.

Unfortunately, our human nature is to make snap judgments about people and to quickly size them up as all good or all bad. We do this not just because we are inhumane and/or ignorant, but, rather, because we are intent on efficiently processing a complex set of environmental stimuli, including all the cues from new people we meet, in order to appraise whether we can predict their behavior or not. This prediction is necessary for our survival, whether it be physical or social. Making perceptual judgments is a deeply ingrained human behavior, but we can take care in guarding against the over-generalizations and stereotyping that produce inaccurate perceptions.

Wilmot (1987) suggests several ways we can perceive others more accurately:

1. We first need to realize that our perceptual biases do not really reflect the other person's qualities as much as they serve us. Knowing this, we then should be willing to modify an initial perception as we obtain additional information about a person. Just because you stereotype a patient as "trouble" because of your past experiences with this "type" of patient does not mean that you can't allow yourself to change that first impression by giving the patient a chance to demonstrate non-troubling behaviors. If we are open to being proven wrong in our initial judgments, we will go a long way toward forming more accurate perceptions.

2. Referring back to the transactional nature of human communication, keep in mind that both participants in a communication interaction are responsible for how they perceive each other and how they communicate together. Most people, on the other hand, tend to see their own behavior as benign or as caused by situational factors (e.g., "I copied the patient's vital signs inaccurately

because I was frantically busy that day"), whereas they view another's behavior as caused by negative qualities in the person, not by the situation or environment. This is known as "fundamental attribution error" (Jones & Nisbett, 1971) and simply means that you over-attribute your own behavior to situational causes and over-attribute someone else's behavior to internal causes (e.g., "Dr. Brown always yells at nurses because he hates professional women"). Again, if you keep in mind that both parties are reacting to and influencing the other, and that all behavior is a product of both situational (external) and personal (internal) factors, then you are not so quick to blame the other and salvage yourself. You acknowledge that *both* of you have inaccurate perceptions and, thus, faulty communication ensues.

3. Recognize that the more time you spend observing and interacting with another, the more accurate your perceptions of him or her will be. More information leads to more accuracy. Of course, we all know this at some level, but we forget to practice it. Our initial perceptions and judgments of an individual get frozen and we refuse to let subsequent contradictory information about the person change them. (Alas, think of how many potentially rewarding relationships we miss out on because of our tendency to discard information that is not congruent with our initial impression).

The ability to accurately perceive both emotions and attitudes improves with time and with increased exposure to a person in different contexts. Allport (1968) claims that a number of personal characteristics are positively correlated with the ability to accurately judge another: personal experience, intelligence, cognitive complexity, self-insight, and social skills. Many of these attributes are learned; they are not innate. Experience is the best teacher, but awareness of what *causes* faulty perceptions can help even the neophyte student of human interaction. And, of course, we add another layer of complexity when we realize that most interpersonal perceptions can't be "checked out" for their accuracy. Sometimes feedback from the one being perceived is the only guide we have as to whether we've misjudged her or him. Occasionally, we have the benefit of getting good advice from an observant friend or coworker, but all these perceptions, whether from the viewpoint of the perceived or the observer, are colored by perceptual biases.

We perceive favorably those people to whom we are attracted more than those we do not find so attractive. While this is only logical, we need to realize that, basically, we like people and find them attractive because: a. they have physical proximity to us; and b. they are similar to us, particularly if they have similar attitudes. (Similar personality traits are not as important to attraction as similar attitudes.) If you are a firm believer in the adage that "opposites attract," you will find the foregoing difficult to accept, but most social science research studies have confirmed that people who are alike and who share the same physical space also share liking. That tendency might make us seem selfish and egocentric. The underlying belief, however, is that we think we will experience more rewarding and less threatening interactions with people who are like us than with people who are different. (This introduces a special problem for health care professionals who must deal with diverse patients from a multiplicity of cultures and backgrounds. More on these problems is discussed in Chapter 4.)

INFLUENCING OTHERS

Many words have been devoted to describe how to win friends and influence people. We especially seem keen on learning what techniques and strategies will work to get our friends and associates to do what we want them to do. In interpersonal communication literature such attempts at influence are usually discussed under the rubrics of power, persuasion, and compliance-gaining. The research in this area, prolific as it has been, unfortunately gives us no recipes, no formulaic strategies for discovering how to control the behavior of others. We realize, of course, that the transactional perspective of interpersonal communication precludes absolute control because both parties exercise mutual influence over the interaction. There are, however, a number of persuasive devices or compliance-gaining strategies that have been found to be effective. Bear in mind that these are highly contingent on the parties involved and on the communication situation. These strategies do not derive from a model of manipulation with one party winning and the other losing; rather, most effective persuasive strategies involve a willingness to try to see another's perspective and a realization that both participants influence each other.

INTERPERSONAL PERSUASION AND POWER

Reardon (1987) discusses interpersonal persuasion as "the intention by at least one communicator to change the thoughts, feelings, or behavior of at least one other person" (p. 125). In contrast to spontaneous interpersonal communication, such intention is manifested in carefully thought-out behavior or strategy. It may even take the form of scripted behavior. (How many of us have mentally practiced our lines for an upcoming encounter with a friend or colleague for whom it's difficult to see things our way?) Some people even memorize a script for any persuasive occasion, refusing to modify their lines for the particular individual or situation. This, of course, is not an effective strategy.

Another way of looking at persuasion is to look at interpersonal power. How much power do you have over another person? McCroskey, Richmond, and Stewart (1986) define this power as "the ability to have an effect on the behavior of another person or group" (p. 186). This ability is moderated by many factors, however, some of which were spelled out by French and Raven (1959) in an article that discussed the five bases of social power: coercive, reward, legitimate, referent, and expert. Let's briefly look at each of these sources of power and examine how they can be used in attempts to exert interpersonal influence.

1. **Coercive power** derives from the persuader's ability to inflict punishment if the persuadee does not comply. For example, years ago it was a common practice to threaten children with an injectable antibiotic if they did not take their oral medicine. This base of power is effective dependent upon a communicator's perceptions of whether any punishment will actually ensue if orders are not followed. (Think of how quickly children can determine whether a parent is only issuing hollow threats.) Another drawback of coercive power is that it does not motivate a person to continue a new behavior or to continue to change an attitude.

Most researchers see coercive power as a last resort measure because the costs, both relationally and practically, are high; however, all of us know communicators who regularly rely on this method to get what they want.

2. **Reward power** is the opposite of coercive power, for it consists of a communicator's perceived ability to reward cooperative behavior. What's the drawback here? If a person is rewarded, he or she will expect subsequent rewards for comparable behavior; otherwise, the lack of such rewards may be seen as punishing. Thus, nurses who offer lavish praise to patients who ambulate without assistance had better be prepared to continually praise these same patients every time they ambulate.

3. **Legitimate power** or "assigned power" derives from the social, occupational, or status role that a communicator plays. If you believe that a hospital administrator has the right to ask you to drive her to work just because she is an administrator, then you are granting that supervisor legitimate power. Because the exercise of legitimate power is often associated with the exercise of punishing behaviors, many people hesitate to use it or to accept it. But frequently our requests for compliance are generated by and legitimated by the professional role we assume. In some instances, we must call on legitimate power to try to persuade a person who otherwise would find no good reason for complying with our wishes.

4. **Referent power** is linked to a person's identification with a specific individual or group that is deemed highly attractive. When an individual whom you are trying to influence perceives you as attractive and wishes to imitate or model your behavior, he or she will often behave in a way that will please you. The person will comply with your requests because he or she wants to be liked by you. (Would that all of our associates perceived us so!) Referent power is potent; it can bring about dramatic behavioral and attitudinal changes. It also works reciprocally because of the transactional communication theory—friends and colleagues model and internalize each other's behavior, building a stronger bond between them.

5. **Expert power** comes from the perception that the persuader is credible—that she or he is competent, knowledgeable, and skilled. This base of power is quite useful since it leads to compliance and also to internalization of a desired behavior or attitude. Again, this type of power is particularly effective in strengthening interpersonal relationships.

McCroskey et al. (1986) point out that one's power bases do not have to be explicitly spelled out in interpersonal communication. In fact, it would seem silly and superfluous for you to say to a patient, "Now, I'm the nurse here, so that legitimates my request to ask you to cooperate while I start your IV. Also, I realize that you like me and want to please me and that you perceive me as rewarding you if you comply." In many instances, appeals to one's power are implicit and, thus, unstated. In any event, it is the other communicator's *perception* of your power and its source that will determine whether a power move is effective or not. Unless you have the ability to constantly wield coercive power and to not be bothered by its aftershocks, you will only be as powerful as your fellow communicator permits you to be. This is the transactional nature of power and is far different from many people's belief that power is a fixed, static, assigned commodity. Rather, the effectiveness of interpersonal power is always a property of the communication transaction or the relationship between people. That means it is constantly in flux.

THEORIES OF PERSUASION

In addition to the perception of interpersonal power as a motivating factor, what other factors do you think cause individuals to be influenced by another? Reardon (1987), Trenholm and Jensen (1988), and others have discussed the predominant theories of persuasion as: *learning theories* (e.g., classical conditioning and operant conditioning), in which people are motivated to learn through reward and punishment; *consistency theories* (e.g., balance theory and cognitive dissonance theory), which predict that we will make our attitudes and beliefs stable and consistent in order to reduce the discomfort of conflicting thoughts, and *social judgment theories* (e.g., latitude of acceptance and latitude of rejection), which emphasize how social norms guide us as to how to respond to a persuasive message.

One of the more compelling theories that explains how humans are persuaded is known as the *ACE Model of Persuasion* (Reardon, 1981, 1984). According to this model, people are persuaded in part by their judgments of how **Appropriate**, **Consistent**, or **Effective** a behavioral option is likely to be. In other words, people either consciously or unconsciously know rules about how a behavior in question might be judged by others (appropriateness); how that behavior fits with one's value system and self-image (consistency); and whether that behavior might lead to a desired outcome or goal (effective). Thus, such social standards or rules are utilized as criteria for rejecting or accepting a persuader's wishes. If the desired behavior is seen by the potential persuadee as socially appropriate, consistent with her or his values and image, and likely to lead to one of the persuadee's goals, then it is far more likely to be accepted.

PERSUASIVE STRATEGIES

We can persuade others because of their perception of our interpersonal power and because we can appeal to their standards of appropriateness, consistency, and effectiveness. With that in mind we can then ask: What are the actual *strategies* for persuasion? And how do we let others know of our power bases without being so explicit that we are counterproductive? Trenholm and Jensen (1988) report that we use self-presentation strategies to inform others that we have persuasive power. Such strategies have been described by Jones and Pittman (1980) as: ingratiation, intimidation, self-promotion, exemplification, and supplication.

These persuasion strategies can be defined as follows:

1. **Ingratiation** relies on the norm of reciprocity, which states that people generally behave toward you as you behave toward them. Thus, if we are amiable and friendly, ingratiating ourselves to others, we can expect like behavior. Of course, this strategy can backfire if your friendly behaviors are perceived as manipulative. One example of such perceived manipulative behavior is the use of insincere flattery to persuade another.

2. **Intimidation**, on the other hand, is the opposite of ingratiation. People who use intimidating strategies are not concerned with whether or not they are perceived favorably by another. In fact,

they frequently engage in aggressive, socially unacceptable behavior to try to control others.

3. **Self-promotion** involves establishing credibility as an expert so that one appears competent and knowledgeable. In fact, self-promoters rely highly on expert power to persuade others. As with ingratiation, however, self-promotion has a downside if the persuader is perceived as a braggart. Since modesty is a highly valued norm in our society, the self-promoter must appear to be somewhat self-effacing while also appearing competent and credible. As you can imagine, this can be quite a juggling act.

4. **Exemplification** means that others perceive you as embodying the values they cherish; thus, they are willing to be persuaded by you. For example, if your actions and demeanor consistently project integrity or other valued attributes, it is difficult for others not to admire you. A nurse who constantly volunteers to work extra shifts on his or her day off to replace personnel who are sick or on leave may be using an exemplification strategy to persuade a supervisor that she or he is dedicated and conscientious. (Again, this strategy can be overdone and can lead to the opposite result—the despised and dreaded brownnoser!)

5. **Supplication** involves the assumption of helplessness. This is probably the least effective self-presentation strategy because if you continually influence others through being so weak and defenseless as to invite protection, then you will find that you are actually losing both your competence and your self-esteem. All of us at one time or another, however, have at least pretended incompetence in order to get another person to feel sorry for us and help us out. Women have been especially susceptible to this strategy because of socialization messages that teach women that they are not as competent as men.

Trenholm and Jensen (1988) remind us that all of these self-presentation strategies can be persuasive when used in moderation and in the right circumstances. When carried to an extreme, however, they can create most undesirable effects. They can dissuade rather than persuade.

COMPLIANCE-GAINING STRATEGIES

What do you think are the actual messages communicators rely on to gain compliance from others? That question is especially salient for professional nurses who constantly seek the cooperation and compliance of colleagues, physicians, other members of the health care team, and, perhaps most importantly, patients. Two researchers, Marwell and Schmitt (1967), are credited with devising the most complete list of compliance-gaining strategies. While we won't discuss all of the 16 methods that they reported, we will note that the 16 methods are derived largely from the five bases of power outlined by French and Raven (1959) and also from Jones and Pittman's (1980) self-presentation strategies. Marwell's and Schmitt's list includes promise, threat, expertise, liking, moral appeal, and altruism as potentially effective strategies.

Other researchers, in a similar vein, discuss *affinity-seeking strategies* (Bell & Daly, 1984), which rely on getting others to feel an affinity or liking for the persuader; *emotional strategies* such as empathy, emotional expressionism, compliment, and insult (Reardon & Boyd, 1986); and *deception strategies* (Knapp & Comadena, 1979), which include white lies, cover-ups, euphemisms, etc., used in an attempt to avoid possible negative reactions to telling the truth. *Comforting strategies* (Burleson, 1984) may be an especially important category of persuasive devices for health care professionals. These strategies involve recognizing another's emotions and life circumstances and taking these into account in utilizing persuasion effectively. Reardon and Buck (1984) and Sullivan and Reardon (1985) found that the level of comfort we give others in a crisis situation, such as a serious illness, actually affects the patient's ability to cope with the condition and even to recover.

You might then ask what factors are relevant to consider in choosing which strategy to use? Trenholm and Jensen (1988) stress that one must take into account situational variables, such as: *intimacy* (the degree of emotional closeness between the communicators); *dominance* (the relative power of each of the communicators); *resistance* (whether you believe the other person will either comply with or resist your request); *rights* (Is the request legitimate?); *personal benefits* (Is the request selfish or altruistic?); and *consequences* (What are the long-term effects of the strategy?) in trying to determine how to get another person to comply with your wishes or requests. Berger (1985) discusses similar factors, but adds: *time available for goal achievement* (you may not have the luxury of considering the consequences of a particular strategy); *degree of success* (how effective has this strategy been in the past?); and *personality* (one strategy might be more comfortable than another, depending upon the persuader's personality).

Which compliance-gaining strategies do you think communicators most often resort to? So far the research is still inconclusive, but Tracy, Craig, Smith, and Spisak (1984) found that more people choose direct, positive approaches than indirect, negative ones. Instead of using threats, for example, research subjects more frequently chose promises ("I'll do something nice for you if you cooperate with me now") and appeals to altruism ("I'd appreciate your doing this as a personal favor to me"). Certainly, these types of strategies don't incur the negative consequences that less positive appeals might. For example, one of Marwell and Schmitt's (1967) strategies termed *negative altercasting* involves persuading someone that only a person with "bad" qualities would fail to comply with the request. You can see how this strategy might prove effective in the short term, but might also have counterproductive long-range ramifications.

Trenholm and Jensen (1988) also discuss the most effective way to structure requests we make of others. Generally, if we establish an acceptable reason for making a request before we actually make it, we will be more persuasive than if we boldly and without rationale ask a person to comply with our request. Convincing another of the need for a requested action or attitude change and asking rather than ordering compliance can prove effective. The face needs of the other must be considered when making a request. Brown and Levinson (1987) describe these needs as wanting to be liked, appreciated, and respected by another; losing face is seen as embarrassing and disruptive to the social interaction. To protect someone's face when asking them to comply with your request requires you to acknowledge the individual's need to be treated with courtesy and respect. We can often "soften" a request, for example, by using the person's name, by greeting her or him courteously, and by taking into account that person's perspective of the situation.

THE POWER OF EMOTION AND FEELINGS IN PERSUASION

One more vital consideration is necessary when trying to persuade another. Most persuasion research has been conducted with the assumption that people are rational, reasonable creatures, who will behave in ways that will maximize their chances of attaining their personal goals. Probably such research has over-relied on cognitive models of behavior and has underplayed the significance of emotion (and irrationality) in persuasion.

Reardon (1987) advises that the power of emotions and feelings must be taken into account when we consider how to influence others. For example, it is very difficult to convince an irritable or angry person to alter an attitude or behavior. In such an instance, trying to change the communicator's feelings might be necessary before attempting to rationally persuade him or her to change anything else. You might ask, how can emotions and feelings be changed? The answer is—with great difficulty! We know, however, that people can be taught to reason about their emotions. For example, one can be encouraged to see that an emotional reaction is unreasonable, or that it is inappropriate, inconsistent, or ineffective (Reardon & Boyd, 1985; 1986).

Further, we can try to alter the belief system that gives rise to certain emotions. For example, if a patient is angry because she or he believes a physician hates all patients, you can try to convince the patient that the physician has a curt manner with patients, but does not really dislike them. Possibly the patient's anger will diminish, if we can tear down her or his faulty beliefs. Frequently, the mere discussion of someone's feelings permits that person to see that such emotions are unwarranted in a particular situation. Empathy and comforting communication play major roles in helping people to see that their feelings can be unproductive in their attempts to secure their goals.

A final word about persuasion: one should keep the Transactional Model of interpersonal communication constantly in mind when planning persuasive strategies. Your choices for a strategy should be shaped by your fellow communicator's choices and by the pattern of interaction you share with her or him. Taking the perspective of the other, realizing why a request for change in attitude or behavior might or might not be palatable, is crucial to effective persuasion.

To recap the highlights of this chapter: the interpersonal influence process is a complex one that requires both cognitive awareness and behavioral adeptness. You have been introduced to some of the major theories that explain how and why humans are persuadable creatures. As nurses, you also need to be cognizant of compliance-gaining strategies and the situational variables that impinge on their effectiveness. Trenholm and Jensen (1988) offer a bit of compact advice on how to persuade: "Competent communicators must be sensitive to the context, to their own self-presentations, and to the target's needs and vulnerabilities. They must then be able to translate this into rhetorically acceptable message forms" (p. 226). This information still does not guarantee that you will win friends and influence people, but not knowing it predicts that you won't.

3

Interpersonal Communication Competence

Now that we are aware of some of the fundamentals of interpersonal communication theory, how can we best put that theory to use in our communication with patients, coworkers, physicians, and other members of the health care team? How can we become competent, that is, effective interpersonal communicators? In this chapter, we will discuss the components of competent interpersonal communication including: using verbal messages effectively; using nonverbal messages effectively; and demonstrating interpersonal relationship skills.

INTERPERSONAL COMMUNICATION COMPETENCE

What does it mean to be a competent interpersonal communicator? First of all, communication competence necessarily includes both cognitive and behavioral abilities; in other words, you must have *knowledge* about the communication process to be an effective communicator, but you must also have the *skills* to enact that knowledge. Most definitions of communication competence propose that competent communicators are able to use their knowledge and their skills in order to attain desired goals. Competence, then, is based upon your ability to define your communication goals for a particular situation, to choose those communication behaviors that will have the best chance of helping you meet your goals, and to enact those behaviors with the realization that the other communicator is trying to get his or her goals met too. Wiemann (1977) summarizes the process as: selecting interactional choices among available communication behaviors, accomplishing interpersonal goals, and recognizing the interpersonal and contextual constraints of communication situations. That is, while you are intent on attaining your own goals, you must always take into account the interpersonal ramifications of doing so. For example, as a nursing professional you may find that shouting at a nursing student helps you get her or his attention, but you may also have to work extra hard following such behavior to win his or her trust and respect. Sometimes we can get what we want only at great expense. As a competent communicator, you must assess how much you are willing to "pay" in the future to get an immediate need addressed. You must always take into account the other's needs and goals as well as the contextual (situational) constraints. An emergency, for example, might necessitate abruptness on your part. In this situation the most competent communication behavior may likely involve a decision to risk *not* being perceived as a kind, empathic communicator. Being aware of that risk and the potentially ensuing costs is part of being a competent communicator.

Unfortunately, there is no laundry list of "competent communication skills" that we should all memorize and pull out for every occasion. The complicating factor about communication competence, as we have seen in Example #1, is that both the situation and the interpersonal consequences shape what will be perceived as appropriate communication. One other caveat about being an effective communicator rests in that word "perceived"; communication competence is assigned or attributed to us by another. We may think that we're competent across audiences and situations, but unless the person with whom we're interacting agrees with that perception, we are not really competent. Also most of us are not so blessed as to be effective communicators in all contexts. Probably, we feel more comfortable in some situations or with some people than with others. The important thing is to learn what behaviors are likely to generate perceptions of competence and to possess the behavioral repertoire to select from these as needed.

INTERPERSONAL COMPETENCE IN NURSING COMMUNICATION

Kreps and Query (1990), in an article linking health communication with interpersonal communication competence, list seven pragmatic communication issues in health care delivery:

1. *Patient compliance*—low levels of compliance have been linked to ineffective health care provider-patient relationships; in turn, noncompliance has been correlated with poor medical outcome, etc.

2. *Miscommunication and misinformation*—ineffective message strategies and failure to seek and to utilize feedback contributes to patients' failure to receive the health care information they need.

3. *Insensitivity* in provider-patient care has been linked to low levels of respect, attempts at relational control, and inaccurate interpretation of nonverbal messages.

4. *Unrealistic expectations and stereotyping* on the part of both patients and providers have led to misinterpretations of each others' needs and inflexibility in role performance. Patients expect medical personnel to be all-knowing; health care providers think patients should be unquestionably compliant—these expectations inevitably lead to disappointment, anger, and resentment.

5. *Lack of interprofessional understanding and cooperation* is a major problem in health care delivery. When health care team members display arrogance and ethnocentrism in their attitudes toward other team members and constantly engage in turf wars, the health care delivery system suffers.

6. *Ethical and moral questions* concerning informed consent, equal treatment and access to health care, confidentiality, and distorting or withholding health information are dilemmas affecting health care delivery. Moral issues involving euthanasia and cultural and religious strictures concerning patient care further complicate the picture.

7. *Dissatisfaction* on the part of both health care personnel and health care consumers is linked to other health communication problems, including failure to express empathy, relational dominance, and dehumanization.

For all of the issues in health care delivery listed above, effective interpersonal communication is critically important. While no communication professional would suggest that competent communication is the panacea for all the health care delivery problems enumerated, we argue that competent interpersonal communication improves the chances for understanding and resolving these problems. The remainder of this chapter is thus devoted to exploring effective verbal, nonverbal, and interpersonal relationship skills and strategies.

INTERPERSONAL SKILLS FOR HEALTH CARE PROFESSIONALS

What are the most relevant communication skills for health care professionals? According to Kreps and Query (1990), numerous research studies have identified these as the abilities to communicate with empathy, to listen nonjudgmentally, to demonstrate interpersonal respect, and to manage interactions. Wilmington (1986) discussed 37 oral communication skills that were identified by nursing supervisors as essential to nurses' communication competence. These were organized into seven top health communication skills, including:

1. giving accurate and sufficient feedback to others
2. listening attentively to others
3. interpreting accurately what others are saying
4. giving clear directions
5. treating others in a professional manner
6. communicating information clearly
7. establishing one's credibility with others

Note how these seven essential skills are dependent upon a transactional perspective of interpersonal communication. Whereas, at first glance, most of these skills might be considered "speaker's" skills (i.e., giving feedback, giving directions, treating others professionally, communicating clearly, and establishing credibility), the exercise of each of the seven skills involves a recognition that the other communicator is as important to the communication process as you are. How we give effective feedback, directions, and information, how we listen and decode accurately, how we treat others professionally, and how we establish credibility are all contingent upon how the other perceives us and what her or his goals are in the communication situation. Thus, competent communication is not just learning, for example, how to use language effectively in order to give clear instructions. It is learning how to select the appropriate vocabulary and sentence structure for the communicator with whom we are dealing. (This concept is explored at length in Chapters 5 and 6, which discuss how to write nursing records for multiple audiences.)

Another study by Morse and Piland (1981) looked at the importance of nine communication skills (advising, persuading, instructing, exchanging routine information, speaking before large groups, communicating in small groups, issuing orders, listening, and managing conflict) in three interpersonal nursing contexts: nurse-nurse, nurse-physician, and nurse-patient interactions. Across all three of these contexts, five skills were consistently listed by nurses as being most essential for competent job performance:

1. listening
2. exchanging routine information
3. managing conflict
4. communicating in small groups
5. instructing

Effective verbal, nonverbal, and relational communication will enable nurse professionals to be perceived as more competent in each of these five essential areas.

USING VERBAL MESSAGES EFFECTIVELY

In discussing verbal communication, we must first take into account that language use or verbal communication doesn't even constitute half the picture when we think of how others perceive our communication competence. Actually, the nonverbal message is equally or more important than anything we say. Furthermore, to attempt to separate out verbal and nonverbal components of messages is somewhat senseless, since both work together to convey meaning. Nevertheless, in the next section of this chapter, we try to distinguish between verbal and nonverbal communication for teaching purposes. Keep in mind when reading both sections that verbal and nonverbal communication are integrally intermeshed.

The verbal messages we send and receive are critical components of the communication process. One of the ways we can improve our chances for accurately encoding and decoding verbal communication is first to realize the distinction between *task* and *relationship messages* (although both task and relationship messages involve nonverbal as well as verbal communication).

Every interaction has two dimensions that are automatically processed by the other communicator as she or he negotiates the meaning of the messages exchanged. These are the task dimensions and the relationship dimensions of a message. Generally, as a nursing professional, you are most interested in the task aspect of a message, the work-centered aspect. For example, in prepping a patient for surgery, your verbal communication to a patient asks that he or she cooperate with the process so that you can perform your job effectively and efficiently.

Example #2

Setting: a preop patient's bedside. The nurse is preparing to give the patient, who is scheduled for colon surgery, an enema.

Nurse Taylor: "Mr. Bush, I need to give you the enema I told you about. So if you'll roll onto your side, I'll put the solution in slowly. When it's all in, I'll take the tube out and you can go into the bathroom."

Mr. Bush: "What if I can't hold it?"

Nurse Taylor: "Just let me know when you're feeling uncomfortable and I'll stop, but remember, it's important that we get your bowels cleaned out before your surgery."

Example #2 demonstrates the task nature of communication—"I'm going to do this and you're going to do that." However, some communication is more informative than task related. How you phrase your request, the actual words you use to give information to the patient and to elicit compliance and cooperation, also conveys relational messages. Note the contrast between these two ways of informing a patient who has never had surgery about the events that precede the induction of general anesthesia.

Example #3

1. *Nurse A*: "The anesthesiologist will place a mask over your nasal and oral cavities in surgery tomorrow, and you will be asked to breathe normally. Just do as she says and you shouldn't have any problems."

2. *Nurse B*: "Ms. Stone, after you get into the operating room, before you are actually asleep, the doctor will place a rubber mask on your face, it may seem a little frightening at first to have your mouth and nose covered by the mask, but it's nothing to be alarmed about. Doctor Swell just wants you to breathe some oxygen and a mixture of gases to help you fall asleep."

In Example #3, Nurse A uses language that is laced with medical jargon and is abrupt and terse; Nurse B, on the other hand, provides information that is more personalized, with lay terms and empathic words that are chosen to comfort as well as inform the patient. Certainly, Nurse B conveys his or her empathy to the patient and assumes the perspective of someone for whom surgery and general anesthesia are both anxiety-producing events. Thus, the relational messages that are received by the patient are likely to be dramatically different for these two dialogues. Nurse A's patient probably perceives that the nurse is performing an obligatory duty, without much feeling for the human being who will be undergoing the operation. Nurse B's language choices signal to the audience that, in fact, the nurse sees this communication event as unique to the patient, Ms. Stone, even though it is likely routine information for the nurse. With these language choices Nurse B communicates empathy and respect for the patient's feelings and condition, and thus establishes relational warmth, support, and rapport.

You may have seen these task/relational aspects of a message demonstrated by some airline attendants who, in giving routine safety instructions at the beginning of a flight, spice up the humdrum seat-belt/oxygen mask information with humor and an idiosyncratic style. Perhaps you appreciate the personalization of the message and the attempt to reduce some fliers' white-knuckled-anxiety by this approach; or, on the other hand, you might find the meshing of humor with safety instructions inappropriate and trivializing. The disparity between Nurse A's and Nurse B's interactions point to a further complexity in task-relational messages: it is essential to know your audience when formulating your message in order to assess how she or he might accept the appropriateness of what you say. Of course, this is easier in one-on-one communication; for group communication, the issue is even more complicated. The important point is that you must combine your task and relational messages in a way that you calculate is most likely to achieve your objectives and also meet the other interactant's goals. Tailoring the message for the other communicator is a critical key to effective communication. (In the case of the flight attendant, she or he can almost certainly count on there being enough passengers who will appreciate her style to offset those who might find it inappropriate!)

Being a competent professional communicator means, too, that you are able to assess those situations in which task is the critical concern and those in which positive relational outcomes are paramount. Not that you don't interweave both task and relationship concerns into every interaction, but frequently a situation will call for focusing more on getting the job done than on soothing feelings and vice versa. Whereas it may be difficult to second guess what encounters call for, what mix of task and relational messages, the experienced competent professional, who is constantly attuned to the other communicator, learns the blend that produces the most effective interaction. The situation, the type of message that needs to be exchanged, and the other communicator all play a part in helping you determine the most successful way to structure a message.

One more caveat about task and relationship messages for nursing professionals: we often hear professionals in all careers excuse their task-dominated communication styles by arguing that it is inefficient to engage in relational "feeling" talk. Surely, health care personnel can rightly claim that the numbers of patients they serve and the complexities of their roles preclude their taking as much time with each patient or coworker as might be needed. We know from previous studies of health care communication, however, that patients judge their satisfaction with health care interactions based on the quality of the interaction more than on the amount of time a health care provider spends with them. Relational talk, messages that personalize the encounter and take into account the patient's feelings, can be quite succinct. For example, Ragan and Pagano (1987) discovered in tape-recorded interactions of a nurse practitioner with female patients that the nurse managed to soothe patients' anxieties about gynecologic exams with a few words. Even something as simple as addressing a patient by her or his name and expressing recognition of his or her anxiety (or pain, or fear, or anger) can communicate a nursing professional's caring and empathy. Of course, the nursing profession has always been heralded for just such qualities, so if you see the previous section as "preaching to the choir," please overlook our communication insensitivity.

CONFIRMING/DISCONFIRMING MESSAGES

Closely related to the task and relationship dimensions of a message are those relationship messages that are seen as confirming or disconfirming. Wilmot (1987) discusses confirmation of the other person as a central contributor to competent communication and to the improvement of a relationship.

What does it mean to confirm someone? We have to notice the other person, true, but we also have to be responsive to her or him through appropriate verbal and nonverbal communication. Because of the norm of reciprocity, which states that people will respond to us with the same behaviors that we display to them, confirming messages often bring about positive responses from the other person. According to Sieburg and Larson (1971), the most effective responses to another are to acknowledge her or him, clarify what she or he has said, give a supportive response, agree about the content of the message, or express positive feelings. In other words, such responses confirm the other person, even without necessarily agreeing with her or him. For example, you can openly disagree with a coworker who says that nursing is a second-class profession, but you can still confirm her or his existence by acknowledging her or his right to that opinion. But if you turn and walk away from a person without saying anything, you are denying her or his existence and thus disconfirming her or him. (This is not to say that disconfirming responses are always inappropriate and always signs of incompetent communication. Any message can be seen as appropriate depending upon the situation, the history of the interactants, etc. But it is important to bear in mind that the relational consequences of continually disconfirming messages can be devastating.)

What constitutes a disconfirming message? Unfortunately, most of us have learned only too well to disconfirm someone through our verbal and nonverbal communication; but we are possibly unaware of some of the messages we send that may be perceived by others as disconfirming. Such categories of messages include: irrelevant, tangential, impersonal, incoherent, incongruent, or impervious messages (Wilmot, 1987). For example, as Satir (1967) has so effectively pointed out in her writings, interactions in which the other doesn't acknowledge our existence or behaves in a completely unexpected manner are invalidating. As Wilmot (1987) explains, "Disconfirming responses usually make the recipient feel confused, unworthy, manipulated, or just plain devalued" (p. 233).

Just because we're careful to avoid disconfirming another in most circumstances does not mean that we won't find ourselves the recipient of disconfirming messages. How do we cope with such messages? Sluzki, Beavin, Tarnopolsky, and Veron (1967) list four strategies for responding to messages that disconfirm us:

1. *Explicit comment*—this involves actually commenting on what the person is doing rather than on the content of the message. For example, if a coworker constantly tries to devalue you, you might respond, "I'm getting irritated trying to talk to you because I think you're always trying to put me down." This may clarify to the other communicator that you see his or her messages as disconfirming. Frequently we don't realize when we are using disconfirming strategies and we need to have these pointed out to us.

2. *Withdrawal*—involves leaving the scene when you can't change the other communicator. Sometimes it's better to withdraw than to try to fight it out and build further tension. A response might be, "We don't seem to be making any progress on solving this problem. Let's try to get back to it later."

3. *Acceptance of only one level of the message*—this is a strategy for confronting messages that you interpret as contradictory or incongruent. Frequently people attempt to manipulate us by saying one thing but meaning another; this is generally accomplished by using nonverbal behavior that contradicts verbal behavior or vice versa. For example, if a patient tells you, "I'm feeling real good today," but says this in a sarcastic tone of voice with his or her eyes downcast, you might respond, "You *say* you feel good, but you sure don't sound like it. What seems to be bothering you?" Or, on the other hand, you may wish to respond to the other level of the message being communicated by stating, "Well I'm sure glad you're feeling so good and sounding so chipper!" Your sarcasm in this case may signal to the patient that you perceive the incongruity between his or her verbal and nonverbal messages. You're onto him or her, in other words.

4. *Counterdisqualification*—sometimes we think we are forced into giving an equally disqualifying response to match the disconfirming message we've received. This is not a strategy that should be abused, but it may be useful occasionally to shock the other into recognizing that there is a problem between the two of you that needs resolving. "I may be late a lot, but at least when I'm here I try to help everybody else out and not just sit at my desk and sharpen pencils all day."

What do we know about language use and the actual word choices of effective communicators? First of all, as has been stressed throughout this chapter, competent communication involves matching diction (vocabulary) and syntax (sentence structure) to the level of understanding you think the other communicator possesses. In other words, as we also point out in chapters 4 and 6, you must know your audience in order to choose how to encode a message that will be clearly understood. While this advice appears so commonsensical as not to merit inclusion, think of how many physicians and other medical personnel you know who always talk "over a patient's head." The use of medical jargon and unnecessarily complicated explanations of medical procedures are constantly being criticized by health care consumers and are, in fact, a primary cause of dissatisfaction expressed by patients with their health care interactions.

In his guide for professional communicators, Hopper (1984) advises about language use: keep it simple; use dialogue; be clear, but not too clear; be relevant; refine your oral skills; learn to talk differently in different situations; and accept different modes of expression. Simplicity is an understandable virtue of spoken communication, especially for health care professionals. The use of dialogue involves the conversational art of involving the other person in the interaction rather than engaging in a monologue. You can help to accomplish this dialogue by asking questions, by listening intently to the other, by paraphrasing the other communicator's ideas and asking for confirmation, and by responding actively to his or her verbal and nonverbal messages.

Being clear without being too clear simply means that you can be informative without giving so much detail that you create disinterest or boredom. We don't, after all, want our patients falling asleep on us while we explain a procedure to them! Being relevant is merely staying on track. In health care interactions, we rarely have the luxury of enough time to deviate from the task at hand, but some of us ramble more than is necessary about irrelevant topics. This does not mean that we should cut out all personal references, stories, anecdotes, jokes, and the like from our interactions; in fact, these generally create rapport and express caring. Being long-winded and indulging in *too* much personal talk, however, also steers the interaction off course and can confuse rather than enlighten the other communicator.

Hopper (1984) notes that professionals can improve their oral communication skills in a number of ways: they can utilize mirrors, cassette recorders, and even videotape, looking and listening for how they might be coming across to others. Both in one-on-one interactions and public speaking performances, these devices have been helpful for many professional communicators. Learning to talk differently depending on the situation is a mark of a competent communicator; keep in mind that flexibility in our communication style is necessary for communicating effectively across a number of different audiences. As you no doubt have already experienced, you simply cannot talk to one patient the same way you address another, and that advice goes for coworkers, physicians, and administrators as well.

Being tolerant of diverse modes of expression is one of the most difficult tasks communicators face. We are bombarded by ways of speaking that we potentially find offensive; speakers who use different accents, who come from different cultural, socioeconomic, and educational backgrounds; who appear sexist or racist or are in some other way prejudiced in their speech habits; who mispronounce words or who use incorrect grammar. Remember that we frequently stereotype speakers according to the ways they speak and that these stereotypes reflect our own prejudices about certain individuals and groups. (It is also wise to keep in mind that others are making assessments about our own speech patterns and may be judging us harshly as well.)

USING NONVERBAL COMMUNICATION EFFECTIVELY

You already know a lot about effective nonverbal communication from having read the previous section on verbal communication. Verbal and nonverbal communication are inseparable to some extent. For example, in order to use task and relationship messages effectively, you rely on nonverbal communication; likewise, you utilize nonverbals when you confirm or disconfirm someone. In fact, nonverbal communication is the channel through which more meaning is expressed than verbal communication; that's the communication fact behind the hackneyed expression, "It's not what you say but how you say it that counts."

Nonverbal communication consists of all those facets of communication that are not contained in the words themselves, including:

1. *vocalics*—vocal features such as voice quality, rate of speech, pitch, loudness, hesitations, and even yawns, and

2. *kinesics*—a broad range of behaviors relying on movement, including:

   a. *postural-gestural behavior*—position and movement of head, limbs, hands, torso, etc.;

   b. *face displays*—facial expressions;

   c. *gaze*—how we use our eyes during interactions;

   d. *proxemics*—space and physical distance between communicators; and

   e. *haptics*—touching behavior.

How do these nonverbal behaviors, when used in various combinations, function to affect meaning? Ekman and Friesen (1969) discussed five different functions of nonverbal behavior:

1. *supporting or complementing the verbal meaning* of an utterance, such as pointing to the bathroom down the hall while explaining to a family member where it is located;

2. *regulating the flow of the interaction,* as in touching someone to get their attention or backing away to end a conversation;

3. *signaling specific meanings understood by members of one's culture,* usually with head, arm, or hand signals; examples are waving, shrugging, or nodding;

4. *conveying idiosyncratic habits,* which bear little relationship to verbal content, such as holding your chin in your hand when in deep thought or fidgeting with a pencil when you talk to someone; and

5. *expressing emotion,* generally through facial expressions, but also through body posture and distance.

Just as you wouldn't expect a native Spanish speaker to understand your verbal messages spoken in English, you also can't expect communicators from different cultural backgrounds to interpret correctly your nonverbal communication. Those of you who have ever spent an extended time in a foreign country know that learning to be fluent in that country's language involves both verbal and nonverbal fluency. Nonverbal signs and signals do not have universal meaning, as many a hapless politician, diplomat, and foreign traveler have painfully experienced. Too, nonverbal behavior as subtle as intonation can dramatically alter a message's meaning; that is why, for example, so many English-speaking communicators have trouble mastering Eastern languages—they may learn vocabulary, grammar, pronunciation, and other aspects of spoken language, but attaining fluency in the nuances of nonverbal communication is all but impossible. Nonverbal language is culturally bound, just as is spoken language.

Grove (1991) lists some important distinctions between verbal and nonverbal communication. An awareness of these is useful in helping us to improve our communication skills.

1. Unlike verbal communication, we are constantly engaged in nonverbal communication in an interaction, even when the other communicator is speaking.

2. We produce nonverbal behavior more spontaneously and more thoughtlessly than verbal communication. For this reason it is more difficult for us to change nonverbal habits that others might find confusing or offensive. This is less true of our facial communication, which we seem better able to control. We are more typically unaware of what our extremities are doing.

3. Because there is no dictionary for nonverbal communication meanings, the nonverbal behaviors that we use are even more dependent on the context for their meaning than is verbal communication. For example, how a person assesses the meaning behind a touch is highly contingent upon the situation and the relationship between the two communicators. Few nonverbal messages have meaning independent of the context, which explains why the accurate interpretation of nonverbal behavior relies upon a highly sensitive communicator.

4. Nonverbal behaviors are always part of a larger pattern; they are integrated with other nonverbal behaviors rather than isolated. For example, if we tried to produce a smile with our mouth and at the same time a frown with our eye and cheek muscles, we would have a difficult task.

5. To summarize the differences, we place more value on verbal cues for objective, denotative information, but place more importance on nonverbal cues for relational, emotional, and attitudinal meanings.

Knowing about the ways in which verbal and nonverbal communication behaviors differ from each other in these essential ways helps us to more accurately read our partner's nonverbal behaviors. How can we become more effective decoders of nonverbal communication? Grove (1991) points to three ways that we can increase our awareness of the meaning of another's nonverbal communication:

1. We can become more attuned to *nonverbal leakage*, those nonverbal cues that the communicator is apparently unaware of that contain information about his or her feelings or attitudes. For example, a patient who is nervously wringing his or her hands communicates to us his or her anxiety, even though his or her words may deny it. Being cognizant of subtle nonverbal behaviors helps us "read between the lines" in interpreting another's emotional state.

2. We can become aware of *clues to deception*—instances in which one's verbal and nonverbal behaviors do not match. Rather than relying solely on a person's words for meaning, we need to note any discrepant nonverbal cues that contradict what he or she says. Markers of deceitful communication have included: decreases in eye contact; increases in foot, hand, and leg movements; increases in idiosyncratic nonverbal gestures that are not correlated to the verbal message; and decreases in the physical directness of the head and shoulders (Knapp, Cody, & Reardon, 1987).

3. We need to focus on the *total context of the interaction* in order to more accurately perceive nonverbal behaviors. We cannot rely on being able to correctly attribute meaning to a single isolated nonverbal cue; for example, a frown might mean disapproval, concern, confusion, anger, or despair, depending on the situation and the complex set of communication cues emitted from a communicator. Important contextual features include the communication setting, what is being said and why, the history of the communicators' relationship, and how a communicator customarily behaves.

In addition, we must be careful not to make judgments based on a single behavior. In determining a patient's mood, for example, we must look at her or his behavior holistically, rather than, say, focusing only on a smile.

Hopper (1984) adds to the above list by advising that we check our perceptions of nonverbal behavior with words. We are often chagrined, for example, to find out that our attributions of someone's emotional state are completely invalid:

> *Nurse*: "Sally, you look so cheerful this morning—did you get good news about your mother?"
> *Sally*: "No, as a matter of fact, I'm feeling really despondent about her, but I decided to try to put on a happy face anyway."

Keep in mind that while all communication is inexact, nonverbal communication can be particularly hard to decipher due to cultural norms that prescribe cheerfulness, modesty, social solidarity, and the like. Trust your intuitions, but also gather enough information to test them out.

INTERPERSONAL RELATIONSHIP SKILLS

We have now looked at some of the verbal and nonverbal components of competent interpersonal communication, but because as nursing professionals you develop relationships with the people you work with and the people you serve, it is also necessary to consider interpersonal relationship competence. Some communicators appear highly skilled at encoding and decoding verbal and nonverbal messages, yet they flounder when they try to sustain relationships of any kind, personal or professional. What constitutes effective relational communication?

Wilmot (1987) speaks of several aspects of relational competence and enhancement; one of the most important of these is conversational management. To effectively manage a conversation, you must first be able to overcome communication apprehension, which McCroskey et al. (1986) call a "fear or anxiety associated with either real or anticipated communication with another person or persons" (p. 47). Whereas everyone faces shyness or reticence about communicating at one time or another, some people are apprehensive across all situations and face devastating interpersonal consequences because they withdraw from social contact. Learning better conversational skills can often help such persons.

Basically, effective conversational skills involve being able to initiate a conversation, maintain that conversation, and terminate the conversation. It sounds easy because we do it everyday. Think again of how difficult it is to begin talking to a stranger or to a person you feel uncomfortable around. Consider how many times you've felt uneasy or awkward as you tried to find polite ways to end a phone call or a face-to-face encounter. Wilmot (1987) believes these interaction management skills are so critical to relational success that he states, "Whether your dyadic partner is your business associate, teacher, friend, lover, relative, or acquaintance, the management of the separate transactions is the single most important determiner of the quality of the relationship" (p. 222).

Particularly because nursing professionals are in the business of caring for people, sometimes for an extended time period, you must be adept at relational communication. If you do not have good interaction or conversational skills, you need to be aware of that fact and work on improving them.

Reardon (1987) adds to the skills needed for effective interpersonal communication such cognitive abilities as empathy, social perspective-taking, and self-monitoring. We all realize why *empathy* or sensitivity to others' feelings is such a vital attribute of nursing professionals. *Social perspective-taking*, on the other hand, involves the ability to understand the alternatives available to other persons in an interaction. Again, this ability hearkens back to the Transactional Model of interpersonal communication discussed in Chapter 2, because social perspective-taking demands that we realize that interaction is a mutual influence process. If you are good at taking the other's perspective, then you are capable of seeing a situation from her or his vantage, determining options available to her or him, and predicting which option she or he is likely to choose. As we discussed in Chapter 2 under the heading of "Persuading Others," social perspective-taking is an especially critical skill when we are trying to persuade someone.

Self-monitoring involves considering the appropriateness of your comments or nonverbal behaviors before you act. Low self-monitors are those who seem to constantly "shoot from the hip" in their interactions without giving much thought to the consequences. As a nurse, you usually cannot afford to be a low self-monitor. High self-monitors, on the other hand, attentively focus on the verbal and nonverbal behaviors of others and use this feedback to guide their own communication behavior—again, such communicators take the transactional perspective in their realization that both interactants affect the success of an encounter. High self-monitoring has also been found to be linked to the ability to persuade others, just as social perspective-taking has.

Two other critical behavioral skills needed for interpersonal relational competence are *behavioral flexibility* and *effective listening* skills. We have intimated throughout this text that effective communicators are flexible communicators: they possess a wide repertoire of behavioral skills and abilities, and they are adept at assessing both interactants' goals and situational constraints in order to select those communication behaviors that promise to be most effective. Further, such communicators realize that alternative behaviors can be performed to attain the same goal. Bochner and Kelly (1974) claim this flexibility to be a vital aspect of communication competence. A nursing professional who is prepared for the unexpected in her or his encounters with patients, physicians, and other members of the health care team is certainly much better equipped to carry off contingency plans than someone who is completely lost when interactions deviate from the anticipated route.

Listening should not be considered a taken-for-granted communication ability in either our personal or professional lives. For example, how many really good listeners do you know? Some researchers have calculated that effective listening takes even more energy than speaking does; perhaps that is why so many of us appear to be lazy listeners. Certainly the ability to listen well is vital to self-monitoring, social perspective-taking, and behavioral flexibility. In fact, you simply cannot find a competent interpersonal communicator who is not also a competent listener.

What can we do to improve our listening skills? First, we must realize that listening is energy-intensive and requires tremendous powers of concentration and attentiveness. Researchers estimate that we spend almost one third of our waking time listening; this is certainly more time than we spend talking, reading, or writing, yet we devote little study or practice time to learning how to listen better. Hopper (1984) lists five steps to more effective listening that can be of great help to nursing professionals:

1. *Prepare for the listening event*—give the other person your full attention, no matter how harried your day is. Try to make the other person comfortable by not appearing distracted and by giving confirming verbal and nonverbal indications that you are really hearing him or her. At least give the impression that you value what is being said to you.

2. *Stay on track*—the key here is to resist distractions by not letting your mind stray to all that you have to do, or to more entertaining thoughts or fantasies. Develop mental discipline by forcing yourself to attend to the listening situation at hand and blocking out all other thoughts. Give every person the gift of your undivided attention and focus for the time you are with him or her.

3. *Listen for central ideas*—since you can think four times faster than the other person can talk, use extra time to summarize and categorize major themes or ideas that the other person is expressing. Sometimes you will need to check out your summary by paraphrasing what you believe the person has just told you and asking him or her to confirm it.

4. *Avoid gut-feeling traps*—don't let what a person says or how he or she says it confirm your prejudices and biases. Try to listen openly and with the attitude that you are speaking to a singular, unique person, not to a cultural stereotype. People often surprise us when we let them. Also, as we discussed in Chapter 2 under "Perception," try not to make quick judgments and appraisals. Hear the other person out. You would want your nurse to do the same if you were the one confined to a hospital bed!

5. *Overcome defensiveness*—listening defensively means that you believe the other person is attacking you and that you must defend yourself. Obviously, this leads to ineffective listening and to

ineffective interpersonal relating in general. Of course, occasionally the other person really is attacking us, but even then, a defensive posture on our part will not help resolve the problem. Defensiveness creates barriers because you are so busy preparing your rebuttal, you refuse to hear the other's feelings and nonverbal cues as well as missing the content of his or her speech.

Now that we've discussed the fundamentals of interpersonal communication, we are ready to begin examining specific examples of verbal and nonverbal communication. As nurses you will frequently need to assess the setting in which you are communicating, and the audience, purpose, and use for the information you want to exchange.

4

Verbal and Nonverbal Communication in Nursing

THERAPEUTIC COMMUNICATION

The term therapeutic communication can have a variety of meanings, but in this chapter we are referring to the nature of health communication that aids in the assessment and treatment of the patient. This form of communication therapy may be achieved through education, information exchange, interviewing, observing, touching, or writing. Too often, we seem to forget the multiple methods health professionals can use to aid ill or concerned individuals in coping with their conditions or fears.

The sense of communication as therapeutic is again dependent on the nature of the interaction and the context in which the communication takes place. For example, a potential audience might consist of a frightened patient who needs only reassurance and a chance to verbalize her or his fears. Another audience might include a group of health professionals who need to exchange information with their colleagues about their mutual frustrations regarding the lack of improvement in a patient's condition. These nurses may benefit from interactions that discuss previous patients with similar illnesses and their responses to treatment. Or perhaps these health professionals merely need a friendly ear in order to vent their disappointment.

As we have stressed throughout this text, the audiences and purposes for communication are as vast as the Milky Way. Your task is to assess what information the person with whom you are interacting needs or expects and try to find a verbal, non-verbal, or written method for effectively communicating that information. For example, a patient with a tracheostomy (who cannot talk) may have just as many questions about his or her illness and treatment as a highly vocal patient. Your task is to provide both patients with a means to communicate with you and then determine a method for addressing their questions and allaying their concerns. For the postoperative tracheostomy patient that method may require a writing tablet or erasable board. For the verbose patient, it may necessitate your interrupting the patient and asking specifically what information the patient wants or just demonstrating your willingness to let the patient talk about her or his fears.

The more you can fine-tune your listening skills, the better you will communicate your interest in aiding the patient and the more heightened your awareness will become of the patient's needs, concerns, and expectations. Improving your listening and observational skills will enable you to better assess a speaker's concerns and expectations and, at the same time, allow you to obtain valuable information about the patient's physical and psychosocial health. Let's look at one example of a nurse-patient interaction and try to evaluate what the patient is communicating and how the nurse is interacting and responding.

Example #4

Setting: Nurse Maxwell has just entered a patient's room. The patient, Ms. Peterson, is nearly 50 years old and was admitted during the night with a history of substernal chest pain. Ms. Peterson is on telemetry. At the time of admission her EKG and cardiac enzymes showed no acute changes. However, it's been nearly two hours since these tests were repeated, and Ms. Peterson has pressed the call light to summon her nurse.

When Nurse Maxwell enters the room, the patient is sitting up in bed, wrinkling the bed sheets in her hands. Ms. Peterson is staring out the window and rarely looks at the nurse. As Nurse Maxwell, who just came on duty, moves about the room verifying the oxygen concentration, checking the patient's vital signs, and making notes on the chart, she rarely looks at Ms. Peterson.

Nurse Maxwell: "What do you need, Mrs. Peterson?"

Ms. Peterson: "I'm not married, my husband walked out on me two weeks ago."

Nurse Maxwell: "Oh, is that why you pressed the call light?"

Ms. Peterson: "I'm concerned about those tests they did a couple of hours ago. Do you know if they were normal, or did I have a heart attack?"

Nurse Maxwell: "I'm afraid only Doctor Bland can give you those results. He should be here in an hour or so. Now, is there anything else you need?"

Ms. Peterson: "Do you think I should call my husband and tell him I'm in the hospital?"

Nurse Maxwell: "I can't tell you what to do. Besides, I thought you said you weren't married?"

Ms. Peterson: "Well, we haven't gone to court yet, but it's only a matter of time. I just don't know if I should call him. (She starts to cry.) It would really hurt if he didn't care that I was sick."

Nurse Maxwell: "Now, now, don't get yourself all upset, men aren't worth it. Get one of those tissues on your nightstand and dry your eyes. I'll be back later to check on you."

Take a few minutes to consider the intricacies of this example. The patient is obviously undergoing some emotional stress; she tries to communicate that to the nurse when she discounts her marriage and then asks for advice about calling her husband. The patient's nonverbal communication also bespeaks her anxiety. She verbalizes her concern about the test results and is obviously restless and avoids eye contact. But instead of Nurse Maxwell making it easier for the patient to communicate by decreasing the distance between them, encouraging eye contact, and changing her positions, she does nothing to alter the patient's nonverbal behavior. In so doing she may communicate an unwillingness to listen and interact relationally with the patient.

In the space below rewrite this scenario. Try to change Nurse Maxwell's verbal and nonverbal communication and see how you think those changes might affect Ms. Peterson's communication.

One of the first clues that a health professional can use when interacting with anyone is to observe the other person's nonverbal behaviors. In Example #4 the patient has communicated her anxiety in a number of fairly obvious ways. First, she called for a nurse, which signals some desire on the patient's part to communicate. Second, Ms. Peterson tried to avoid eye contact, and she used her hands to display her agitated state.

An effective communicator can use these simple observations to help determine how to interact with someone. If Nurse Maxwell had closely observed the patient's nonverbal signs and concluded that the patient needed some reassurance, the nurse might have positioned herself between Ms. Peterson and the window, thus communicating nonverbally her willingness to listen and exchange information with the patient. If the nurse had noticed Ms. Peterson's signs of apprehension, she might have asked the patient directly if she were anxious and how Nurse Maxwell could help alleviate Ms. Peterson's concerns. Perhaps, if Nurse Maxwell had touched one of Ms. Peterson's hands while she talked with her, she could have signaled her willingness to participate in a meaningful dialogue. And, finally, if Nurse Maxwell had used eye contact to reassure her patient, she might have provided the impetus Ms. Peterson needed to discuss her physical and psychosocial concerns.

Nurse Maxwell, as so frequently happens to busy health professionals, seemed in a hurry to solve whatever immediate problem caused Ms. Peterson to press the call button. However, if you approach a patient with the attitude that you are only available to aid in correcting an immediate problem, you may miss an opportunity to gain valuable information about the patient's physical and psychosocial condition, information that cannot be supplied in a "quick-fix" mode.

Example #5

Let's go back and rewrite Example #4, but this time Nurse Maxwell has entered Ms. Peterson's room, taken a minute to observe the patient's nonverbal behavior, and then moved next to Ms. Peterson's bed, between the patient and the window, and has lightly placed her hand atop Ms. Peterson's.

Nurse Maxwell: "Hi, is it Ms. or Mrs. Peterson?"

Ms. Peterson: "I guess it's Ms., my husband left me two weeks ago."

Nurse Maxwell: "Oh, I'm sorry. That must have been really hard on you."

Ms. Peterson: "Devastating. I don't think I'll ever get over it."

Nurse Maxwell: "Relationships are so difficult. Listen, my name is Sally Maxwell and I'm going to be your nurse for the next eight hours. I noticed your call light was on, are you having any chest pain, or did you need something?"

Ms. Peterson: "I'm just dying to know about those blood tests and that cardiogram they did a couple of hours ago. I'm scared to death that I've had a heart attack, but nobody around here seems to care."

Nurse Maxwell: "We care! Doctor Bland has you connected by this little box to a cardiac monitor and someone is watching your heart pattern constantly. Plus, the nurses have been in here at least every hour checking on you and getting your vital signs." (The nurse moves closer to the patient and smiles.) "I haven't seen the report, but Dr. Bland should be here in just a few minutes to make rounds, and he'll be able to answer your questions. I can tell you that your heart pattern and your vital signs haven't changed since you came in—that's good news."

Ms. Peterson: "Thank you, I know I'm being silly, but I'm just so upset. I didn't mean anything."

Nurse Maxwell: "It's o.k. It sounds like you've got good reasons to be upset. Are you having any pain right now?"

Ms. Peterson: "No."

Nurse Maxwell: "Are you having any trouble breathing or shortness of breath?"

Ms. Peterson: "No. I think I'm just scared."

Nurse Maxwell: "I can understand that. It sounds to me like you've had a pretty rough couple of weeks. When did you first notice the pain in your chest?"

Ms. Peterson: "A couple of weeks ago, but it got worse last night."

Nurse Maxwell: "What were you doing last night when it started hurting?"

Ms. Peterson: "I was just talking on the phone."

Nurse Maxwell: "Huh, I get pains sometimes when I get my phone bill, but usually not when I'm talking on the phone. (They both laughed.) Did someone say something that upset you?"

Ms. Peterson: "My husband. He told me he was moving in with his secretary and he didn't love me anymore."

Nurse Maxwell: "That must have hurt a lot. Did you tell Dr. Bland about the call?"

Ms. Peterson: "I told him I was on the phone when the pain started, but he didn't ask who I was talking to."

Nurse Maxwell: "Did your chest pain start a couple of weeks ago before, or after, your husband moved out?"

Ms. Peterson: "After. It was the first night I tried to sleep in that big bed by myself."

The differences in this interaction, both in the nurse's communication and the patient's, are obvious and illustrative. Dyadic communication is greatly influenced by the willingness of both interactants to listen, observe, and participate in an exchange of information. In Example #4 neither of the participants appeared aware of the need to demonstrate their interest in communicating. Obviously, both of the interactants had a reason for communicating, but neither of them supplied the impetus to promote effective communication and the exchange of information. However, in Example #5, Nurse Maxwell's response to the patient's nonverbal and verbal communication allowed for a significant exchange of information. The nurse learned much more about the patient's physical and psychosocial condition, and the patient learned that the nurse was willing to listen and to be compassionate and optimistic about her condition.

Remember that your willingness to observe and listen will greatly enhance your ability to communicate with any audience and improve your chances of participating in therapeutic communication interactions that benefit all of the interactants. Some settings, however, are much more difficult to control, and your ability to provide social support via your communication may be compromised by the context in which that communication occurs.

SUPPORTIVE VERSUS AUTHORITATIVE FUNCTION

Your communication behaviors, language choices, and nonverbal actions frequently determine whether you will be perceived by a patient as a supportive health care professional or as an authoritarian dictator who is more interested in her or his demands than in the needs of the patient. All too often an individual's communication behaviors are the result of a previous experience with a similar setting or context, rather than ensuing from a calculated assessment of the present situation and the needs and expectations of the other interactant.

Let's look at how the context of a particular setting may influence the communication behaviors of both interactants.

Example #6

Setting: An emergency room in a rural hospital. It's nearly midnight and an inebriated, 25-year-old man is pacing around the small E.R., dripping blood from his lacerated left hand. The nurse, who is waiting for the doctor to arrive from home, wants to clean the wound and stop the bleeding; however, she is standing at a small sink across the room from the patient and is practically shouting as she speaks.

Nurse Juarez: "Mr. Stinson, your hand is bleeding and I can't get it stopped if you won't cooperate and come over here and sit down."

Mr. Stinson: "Either you get a doctor in here right now and fix my hand or I'm going back to that bar and get even with the jerk that cut me."

Nurse Juarez: "Look, I'm the nurse here and I'm telling you that you're losing a lot of blood. Now if you don't want to bleed to death, please get over here and sit down!"

Mr. Stinson: "Up yours!"

Nurse Juarez: "If you don't sit down, I'm going to call the police."

Mr. Stinson: "If you don't stop bossing me around and get my hand fixed, I'm going to call my lawyer."

Nurse Juarez: "Mr. Stinson you're acting like a spoiled child. Now, I'm waiting for you to start acting like an adult and sit down so I can stop that bleeding. Remember, the sooner you start to cooperate and we get that bleeding stopped and your hand cleaned up, the sooner you can get on your way."

Please answer the following questions about the interaction in Example #6.

1. Circle the type of power bases you think the nurse in this example is attempting to use in her efforts to influence the patient's behavior. (Refer to Chapter 2 for the definitions of the five power bases.) [circle as many as you think apply]

    Coercive Power   Reward Power   Legitimate Power

        Referent Power   Expert Power

2. Explain your reasons for choosing the power base(s) in response to question #1.

_____

_____

_____

_____

3. How would you have dealt with Mr. Stinson if you were the nurse in this example? (Be specific and explain the reasoning behind your communication behaviors.) [Obviously, quitting your job or ejecting him from the E.R. are not acceptable responses]

_____

_____

_____

_____

_____

Example #6 illustrates one of the most difficult and frustrating dyadic relationships nursing professionals encounter. The patient, who is both in need of your services and cognitively unstable due to his intoxication, creates a communication dilemma. The nurse in Example #6 attempts to deal with the patient by using a variety of power bases to try to persuade the patient to comply with her requests. The nurse tries to coerce the patient by threatening him with calling the police. She tries to use both legitimate and expert power by reminding him that she is a nurse and he is in need of emergency care. She attempts to use reward power by promising that he'll stop bleeding and get to leave quicker if he cooperates. And, finally, she uses referent power by comparing his behavior to that of a spoiled child and to promising that his cooperation will demonstrate an adult-like role in his care.

What makes this all-too-typical E.R. interaction so ineffective? Obviously Nurse Juarez is dealing with a belligerent patient, who, instead of cooperating and trying to assist her in the treatment of his lacerated hand, is making her job almost impossible. In order for you to experience some of the difficulties in dealing with communication problems like those presented in this example, rewrite the dialogue, but begin by only rewriting Nurse Juarez's portion. Feel free to use both verbal and nonverbal communication to assist you. After you rewrite the nurse's dialogue, keeping in mind the Transactional Model of communication we discussed in chapters 2 and 3, rewrite the entire dialogue.

You have just discovered why the health care arena will never be completely automated. Human beings are complex creatures, and, as such, our interactions require sophisticated, rapid processing of information in order to achieve a satisfactory outcome. In Example #6, we can all agree that the interaction is not acceptable from either the nurse's or the patient's viewpoint. It is true that we could be judgmental and decree the patient's self-induced, altered mental condition as the cause of this unacceptable interaction. As you know, however, there are going to be numerous patients with alterations in cognition that cause them to respond in similar ways. These behaviors may be the result of trauma or disease and therefore cannot be so cavalierly categorized as, "It's the patient's fault. There wasn't anything I could do." While it is often difficult, and occasionally impossible, to deal with confused or irrational patients, your responsibilities necessitate that you try.

Let's look at your rewrite of Example #6. One aspect of the original dialogue that is disturbing is the nurse's treatment of the patient as though he were a child. She attempts to control his behavior by assuming an authoritarian role. Her language choices, therefore, put him on the defensive and are counterproductive for both interactants. If you changed the nurse's dialogue so that she used language that empowered the patient with adult choices rather than mere responses to the nurse's demands, then Mr. Stinson is given an opportunity to achieve an objective that he chose himself. That is, he can get his lacerated hand repaired. Frequently, health care professionals forget that patients, even inebriated patients, still have a right to make choices about their medical care. This right can often be provided by reminding a patient such as Mr. Stinson that he or she chose to come to the E.R. for treatment and that the treatment requires certain behaviors by both the patient and the nursing professional. The task dimension of the message the nurse is communicating to the patient is paramount to the health professional's objective because this scenario occurs in an emergency setting, and Mr. Stinson is both angry and inebriated. The possibility also exists that Mr. Stinson may have additional injuries that are not as obvious as his bleeding hand. Therefore, it is imperative that the relationship dimension of the interaction ("I'm here to help you, but I need your cooperation") is communicated as well. The nurse's dialogue in Example #6 demonstrates language choices and an interpersonal communication style that are totally task-centered. As a result, the nurse does not calm the patient's anxieties, but exacerbates them. The conversation deteriorates to shouting and threats by both interactants, while the basic objective for both parties—treatment of the patient's wounds—is undermined.

In addition to changing her language choices, you might have altered the nurse's nonverbal behaviors as well. For example, you might have changed the nurse's tone of voice from authoritative and loud to soft and empathic. You might have included an attempt at eye contact with the patient. And even though touch might seem too dangerous in this context, the nurse could have offered the patient a sterile gauze pad and encouraged him, not commanded him, to place it with gentle pressure on his wound. In this type of volatile setting, as in most communication situations, the nonverbal messages you communicate frequently carry more meaning than anything you might verbalize. You may recall that the norm of reciprocity that we discussed in Chapter 3 predicts that people will behave toward us as we behave toward them (i.e., shouting begets shouting, demands illicit threats, empathy and concern generate cooperation). In Example #6 it would not be surprising to find that both the nurse and the patient claim the other's behavior *caused* their behavior. So, Nurse Juarez would blame the patient's behavior for her communication style, and the patient would respond that he was hostile because the nurse wanted to boss him around rather than help him.

If we go back to the opening lines of Example #6, it is possible that the entire dialogue might have changed if Nurse Juarez's response to the patient's belligerence, "either you get a doctor in here, or," had been a calm, reassuring tone of voice and a sterile pad for him to place on the wound. Perhaps, she could have responded to his demands by explaining, "I've called Doctor Winger. He only lives about three or four minutes away. I need to clean up that cut before he gets here, but I'm going to need your help in getting the bleeding stopped. We need to soak it. Would you be more comfortable sitting down, or would you like to stand and I'll put the basin on the counter next to you?"

In this rewrite of a portion of the dialogue from Example #6, the nurse has empowered the patient by informing him of her actions in notifying the doctor, by approximating the amount of time it will take for the physician to arrive, and by communicating what needs to be done to begin the treatment. By using the word "we," she assures that the patient understands that he is involved in his treatment decisions and not merely a pawn controlled by an authoritarian health care team. Finally, the nurse uses relational communication and demonstrates her compassion and concern when she asks the patient to decide where to position himself so he'll be comfortable.

Of course you realize that any psychologically impaired patient, whether the impairment results from some type of drug abuse, trauma, or disease, may be incapable of rational discourse, and the nurse may be left with no other option but authoritative and commanding language choices and behaviors. And, if all else fails, a nursing professional may require the assistance of some type of security force for his or her own protection, as well as for the protection of other patients and staff. Effective communication relies on both participants' willingness to cooperate in attaining mutual goals and objectives. Your ability to communicate your support and assistance to patients and their families will increase the likelihood of your success in achieving effective communication and positive results in the care and treatment of patients.

NURSE-PATIENT INTERVIEWS AND RELATIONAL DEVELOPMENT

One of the many important roles of nursing professionals is that of interviewer. The Joint Commission on Accreditation of Healthcare Organizations (1991) requires that nurses assess, "each patient's need for nursing care related to his/her admission" (p. 131). These assessments are typically done through interviews and physical examinations. An example of a nurse-patient interview follows:

Example #7

Setting: A patient's room. The patient, a 47-year-old man, is in bed. The nurse, a 26-year-old man, is standing next to the patient's bed, holding a clipboard and reading off it. The nurse rarely looks up from the papers on the clipboard.

Nurse Glare: "I'm here to ask you some questions about your illness."

Mr. Motley: "I just got finished answering the doctor's questions, can't you ask her?"

Nurse Glare: "No sir, I can't. This isn't my idea, the hospital makes us do this, so try and bear with me and we'll get done just as quickly as possible."

Mr. Motley: "Well, let's get started. My side is killing me, and they said that shot would help, but so far it hasn't done a thing."

Nurse Glare: "When did your pain start?"

Mr. Motley: "About an hour ago."

Nurse Glare: "Did you notice any blood in your urine?"

Mr. Motley: "No."

Nurse Glare: "Oh, I thought they said you had blood in your urine."

Mr. Motley: "The doctor, she said there was blood in it when they looked with the microscope."

Nurse Glare: "Oh. Have you ever had cancer?"

Mr. Motley: "No."

Nurse Glare: "Diabetes?"

Mr. Motley: "No."

Nurse Glare: "A heart attack?"

Mr. Motley: "No. Listen, my side is hurting. Can we do this later, or can you leave that paper and I'll answer the questions when I'm not hurting so bad?"

Nurse Glare: "I've only got a few more and I couldn't leave this paper. Besides, I get off duty in 20 minutes, and I've got to get this done before I go. How about ulcers?"

In order for nursing professionals to conduct a satisfactory interview, both the interviewer and the interviewee should be relaxed and comfortable with discussing highly personal information. The interviewer needs to be observant and attentive to the interviewee's nonverbal behaviors, as well as her or his verbal communication. While it may be necessary to have a list of questions, an interviewer should make every effort to memorize the list and only refer to it on rare occasions. If you must write down the interviewee's responses, make short, quick notes that you can use later as a reminder of the entire response. In addition, avoid writing down every response; rather, make it a point to note only the important positive responses so that a lack of notation means that you can fill-in a negative response at a later time after you've completed your interview. This lack of reading and writing frees you and allows you to maintain eye contact with the patient and observe her or his behaviors and responses. If you are busy reading the questions or writing down detailed responses, you may miss a subtle nonverbal or a quiet verbal response that could place a totally different meaning on a patient's answer. For example, if you asked a patient if he or she had children, and the response was no, you would miss the important significance of a frown or a tear if you were writing the response and reading the next question, instead of observing the patient.

In addition, never forget that your nonverbal behaviors communicate a breadth of information to the interviewee about your credibility, compassion, and professionalism. Standing over someone as you relentlessly grill them with one question after another makes you appear more like a police detective than a caring, compassionate nursing professional.

For a few minutes forget that you are, or are about to be, a nurse. Instead, become the patient in Example #7, and, in the space that follows, write down your thoughts, feelings, and responses to the nurse's actions, words, and implied attitudes. In other words, if you were Mr. or Ms. Motley, in pain and recently interviewed by a health professional, how would you respond to an interviewer like the nurse in Example #7? (Be specific and try to explain the reasons for your response.)

You may have been surprised by the anger and frustration you felt as you tried to communicate your pain to the nurse. Patients are too frequently treated like prisoners, rather than health consumers. This inversion of the patient-provider relationship occurs when an individual's suffering and illness is undervalued or ignored, and the needs and requirements of health care professionals takes precedence over the needs and requirements of the patient.

If we wanted to improve the interaction that occurs in Example #7 and make it a more effective and successful communication exchange, we could start by changing several nonverbal behaviors. First, the nurse could enter the patient's room, after knocking, and explain to the patient that the hospital needs additional information about the patient's illness or injury and his previous medical history. It would be helpful if the nurse provided the patient with an approximation of the time it will take to conduct the interview. If the patient agrees, then the nurse could pull a chair up to the patient's bedside and sit near the patient, at eye level, and proceed with the interview. If the patient is reluctant to proceed at that time, the nurse could explain the importance of the interview to the patient's treatment and request the patient's cooperation in that treatment.

However, if the patient is in pain, partially impaired because of narcotics, illness, or injury, then the nurse should withdraw and either interview a family member or wait to do the interview at a later, more favorable time. Try to remind yourself that the interview should be done at the patient's convenience whenever possible and not at the nurse's.

The issue of credibility again enters into this discussion. Your credibility as a competent, compassionate nursing professional is certainly called into question if you proceed with a lengthy interview of an ill patient. Again, ask yourself how you would feel if you were in pain and the nurse were more concerned about getting the paperwork done than in alleviating your suffering. Relationally speaking, such behaviors, as witnessed in Example #7 above, are counterproductive and only serve to detract from a positive nurse-patient relationship. Consequently, such behaviors make effective patient-nurse communication almost impossible.

Whenever the interview does take place, you should attempt to sit down next to your patient, to be on the same level with her or him, and thereby demonstrate your willingness to decrease the authoritative aspect of your relationship. Try to use eye contact at all times. Ask general questions that allow the patient to respond more fully instead of specific questions that only elicit yes or no answers. For example, instead of "Did you notice any blood in your urine?," you might ask, "Have you ever noticed any blood in your urine, or has your doctor ever told you that you have blood in your urine?" This latter question allows a patient to discuss not only the current reason for hospitalization, but also previous episodes of hematuria. Questions such as "Have you ever had any kind of heart trouble?" or "Do you have any problems with your bowels?" rather than specific questions such as "Do you have a heart murmur?" or "Have you had a heart attack?" allow a patient to discuss a wide range of problems. You can always ask specific questions to clarify a patient's response, but if you start out too specifically, you might miss some valuable information. (Review Ms. Peterson's responses in Example #4.)

Why can't a patient fill out at least a portion of the assessment questionnaire? Too often health care professionals assume an authoritative role and disenfranchise patients. If it makes it easier on the patient to complete the form at a later time, and it will not interfere with her or his care, why shouldn't patients be allowed to complete the form. It offers them a bit more privacy and control, and such an action demonstrates your willingness to cooperate with the patient in affecting the least painful course of treatment.

Finally, it is important to remember that the interview and assessment of a patient is frequently the first, and sometimes the longest, single contact a nursing professional has with a patient. The relationship you forge and nurture during that interview will play a major role in the cooperation and communication that exist in the days and weeks of the patient's hospitalization. The nurse in Example #7 has done little to foster a satisfactory relationship and, consequently, future nurses will have to demonstrate that their attitudes, behaviors, and goals are different than Nurse Glare's in order to communicate effectively with Mr. Motley. Your relationship with a patient is determined by two major factors: the way you communicate your concern and credibility and the patient's experiences with previous nursing professionals. You cannot change what has taken place prior to your interactions with the patient, but you can demonstrate, in both your verbal and nonverbal communication, your desire to cooperate with the patient in order to achieve her or his health care goals.

SPECIAL PROBLEMS IN NURSE-PATIENT COMMUNICATION

We have already touched on a few of the special problems you may encounter in your attempts to communicate effectively with patients. We discussed the problems inherent in trying to communicate with cognitively impaired individuals. Obviously, patients who are in pain or who are anxious about their conditions are more difficult to communicate with than individuals who are painless and worry-free. But what about patients who are deaf, blind, or from different cultures and ethnic backgrounds. These patients create enormous challenges, in terms of effective communication, for nursing professionals. It is beyond the scope of this text to offer specific solutions to many of these challenges, but we can point out a few obvious actions that can assist you in communicating with patients who require special consideration.

Blind patients use their sense of hearing to assist them in observing, but they also rely on their sense of touch. So you need to be willing to use a variety of nonverbal behaviors to assist you in communicating with blind individuals. For example, you may want to draw a picture in a blind patient's hand to help him or her visualize whatever you are describing. Sometimes it is especially helpful to let the patient touch and feel something before proceeding with a treatment or a test. If you want a patient to move from a bed to a stretcher, you could ask the patient if he or she wants to feel the dimensions of the stretcher before asking her or him to move on to it. You can allow patients to touch a pill or capsule before swallowing, rather than dropping an unknown object into their mouth. Try to use language that is much more descriptive than usual—remember, you are that person's eyes and, consequently, you need to communicate how something appears in order for the patient to perceive what it looks like.

Similarly, a deaf person can use her or his eyes to assist her or him in communicating. You can obviously help that individual by having writing materials at the bedside and talking slowly with your mouth in full view of the patient. In addition, patients with hearing, speaking, or visual deficiencies should have their charts clearly marked, so that all health care professionals are aware of the needs of the patient prior to their first encounter.

Patients with aphasia or dysphasia create a slightly different problem for nursing professionals. If the patient can write, if he or she has no paralysis, then you can improve the patient's communication effectiveness by supplying him or her with a note pad or erasable board. Remember to leave a bell or call light within easy reach of the patient so that help or assistance can be quickly summoned. Try to avoid rushing a patient with a speech disorder. Frequently, well-meaning health care professionals try to finish sentences, guess the meaning of phrases, etc., for patients with speech disturbances. While the intention of the listener may, in fact, be to aid the speaker, the listener, instead, is often perceived as rushing the speaker or lacking the compassion to allow the speaker to complete a sentence or phrase without interruption.

It is also important to note that health care professionals frequently err by treating patients with hearing, visual, or auditory disturbances as though they are children. In fact, these patients often require a little different approach than non-impaired patients, but they should still be treated with respect and dignity and as adults. For example, you would never think of walking into a sighted or normal hearing patient's room and without warning touch that person. Yet, health care professionals often do exactly that to visual- and hearing-impaired patients. Imagine, if you will, how you would feel if you were sick and in a strange bed and suddenly you feel a stranger's hand on your body. That kind of well-intentioned violation contributes to communication problems between health care professionals and impaired patients. If you walk in a patient's room and he or she is blind, speak to that person before you approach too quickly. Let him or her know who you are and why you are approaching. It is a good rule to ask a blind person's permission to touch or physically assist her or him. Don't assume that someone's blindness gives you permission to assist or touch the person. You wouldn't appreciate such an action, and neither will they. If you enter the room of someone who is hearing impaired, move into her or his visual field at a distance and only move closer when it is obvious that she or he recognizes you. If a hearing-impaired patient is asleep, you are faced with a more difficult communication situation, but standing at the foot of the patient's bed and gently moving the bed until the patient awakens is one way to communicate your presence without violating the person's right to privacy.

Patients who are from different cultures or ethnic backgrounds than you present an additional communication problem. As we discussed in Chapter 3, not only is verbal communication frequently impossible because of language barriers, but often, nonverbal behaviors have markedly different meanings when communicating with people from other cultures. For example, it may be inappropriate in certain cultures to have a health professional of the opposite sex touch a patient. A simple nonverbal response, such as smiling at a stranger, may be unthinkable in certain cultures. In addition, some patients may be unable to talk about certain anatomical aspects of their illness because it is forbidden in their cultures. Or some cultures may be so repressive that discussions of impotence or orgasm may be taboo. It is only through education and inquiry that you will learn more about the interethnic and intercultural communication differences of your patients. Remember, it is your responsibility to find an effective means to communicate with patients. Consequently, you may have interactions that require you to use an interpreter, obtain information about the patient's customs and culture, or gain assistance from the patient's family. Whatever means you choose, try to always maintain your respect for the patient's dignity and culture, and it will be easier for you to obtain her or his cooperation.

Another area of patient-nurse interaction that is frequently problematic for nurses is patient compliance. Part of your role as a health care professional requires that you gain your patients' trust and their families' confidence so they can cooperate with and assist you in the patient's treatment. One way to gain compliance is through developing positive relationships with patients and their families. A patient who trusts you will generally comply with your requests. If, however, patients do not trust you or if they feel that you are not interested in their welfare, you will have a difficult, if not impossible, time getting them to comply. The patient in Example #4 is a good model of the difficulties you may encounter in getting a patient to comply with your wishes. The reverse is also true. If you demonstrate your care and concern as well as your compassion and interest in the patient's well-being, most patients will comply with your requests. Conflict resolution, however, is not the only difficult type of nurse-patient communication.

In order to gain the patient's compliance you should try to use language and nonverbal behaviors that demonstrate your competency and credibility as well as your desire to do what is best for the patient.

Example #8

Setting: A patient's room, the female patient is 62 years old and in the hospital for treatment of a bleeding ulcer. The nurse enters the room just as the patient is about to bite into a hamburger that she has smuggled up to her room.

Nurse Weave: "Hello Ms. O'Toole, you must be feeling better today?"

Ms. O'Toole: "I guess I will be as soon as you leave me alone, so I can eat this burger."

Nurse Weave: "Well, I could leave you alone, but then I wouldn't be doing my job. You see, I'm supposed to teach you what's healthy for you to eat and what isn't. As it turns out, that hamburger isn't so good for your ulcerated stomach."

Ms. O'Toole: "I see. So, you want to steal my lunch, is that it?"

Nurse Weave: "No, I'm afraid not. You see, they assigned me to you because they knew I could teach you all about how to eat with an ulcer."

Ms. O'Toole: "And why might that be? Are you a cook or a dietitian?"

Nurse Weave: "Neither, I'm just a woman like you, with an ulcer."

Ms. O'Toole: "Go on with you."

Nurse Weave: "I'm not going to lie to you. I tend to worry a bit too much and that seems to be bad for my stomach lining."

Ms. O'Toole: "What's the stomach lining got to do with it?"

Nurse Weave: "Well, it just so happens that ulcers form when stomach acid increases because of stress or too much fried food or alcohol. Even aspirin can aggravate it."

Ms. O'Toole: "So this hamburger is going to make my stomach hurt worse because there'll be more acid in there."

Nurse Weave: "Now you're an ulcer expert too. Do you think the burger is worth the pain and maybe more bleeding?"

Ms. O'Toole: "You're a sneaky one, you are. Now my burger's cold. So tell me, what do you eat instead of hamburgers?"

In Example #8 Nurse Weave uses self-disclosure to gain the patient's trust and eventual compliance. Self-disclosure is one method that works well in gaining people's trust, but never lie in order to try to convince patients. They'll figure you out every time, and that can cause a marked distrust. If Nurse Weave had not been a victim of ulcer disease herself, what other methods might she have used to gain Ms. O'Toole's trust and enhance her compliance?

_____

_____

_____

One method Nurse Weave could have used is a similar story about a relative or a friend with ulcer disease. If that didn't apply, she could describe a previous patient's experience with ulcer disease. All of these examples do essentially the same thing—they help to establish Nurse Weave as an "expert," but not in the distanced "I learned it in school" sense, rather in the "I'm one of you, I've been there" sense. A totally different approach would have consisted of explaining the way ulcers form and are effected by acid and internal and external factors—

an attempt to motivate the patient by education and encouragement. Again, the nurse can be seen as an expert, but the patient still has the power to make her own choices. It will not do the patient or the nurse any good for the nurse to run across the room, steal the sandwich, and chastise the patient as though she were a 4-year-old child. Adults generally respond best to being treated as adults, so that when they are educated about something, if they believe the educator, find her or him a credible and professional person, then they are more likely to follow her or him suggestions and recommendations.

Compliance, then, results from trust, education, and explanation. Seldom do health care professionals gain patient compliance by threats or fear tactics. Ask yourself this question: Do I respond better to someone telling me not to do something, or when they explain that I can do it, but my actions may very likely result in injury to myself or others? If you're like most people, you will frequently rebel against the commanding approach, but if you trust the educator, you will very likely be swayed to alter your behavior by a speaker who explains the risks and the reasons for avoiding certain behaviors.

Another area of nurse-patient communication that is a difficult aspect of professional nursing is your role in conflict resolution. Occasionally, you will find yourself in the uncomfortable position of playing referee. Sometimes it will be a disagreement between patients and their families or patients and physicians, but one of the most difficult conflicts to help resolve is one between a patient and a colleague. You run the risk of alienating either your patient or your peer and neither of those two alternatives is acceptable. Let's look at an example of a nurse-patient conflict and an attempt at achieving a resolution.

Example #9

Setting: The E.R. of a large metropolitan hospital. Nurse Stanley is working, and Nurse Frost is the charge nurse. A young female patient, age 18, is arguing loudly with Nurse Stanley.

Nurse Stanley: "The doctor has ordered these X-rays, he wants to find out what's causing your pain."

Ms. Hellman: "I don't want any X-rays. I just want something to make this pain go away."

Nurse Stanley: "Well, we can't give you anything for your pain until we know what's causing it. Now, why don't you lie back and let me take you to X-ray and then we'll see about getting you something for your pain."

Ms. Hellman: "I'm not going to let you shoot me full of radiation."

Nurse Frost: "Hi. Can I be of any help."

Ms. Hellman: "Yea, you can get rid of this nurse. She won't listen to anything I have to say."

Nurse Stanley: "Doctor Marquez ordered an IVP. He wants to see if she has a kidney stone. I've tried to explain that to her, but she just refuses to cooperate. All she's interested in is getting some pain medicine."

Ms. Hellman: "Hey, I'm no druggie, but this damned thing hurts and no one seems to care."

Nurse Frost: "Do you know what a kidney stone is?"

Nurse Stanley: "I explained it to her and gave her a handout that describes it in detail, but she just won't listen to reason."

Ms. Hellman: "That's your reasoning. Why don't you lay here awhile, with your side hurting, and see how well you listen."

Nurse Frost: "I understand that you're hurting and so does Nurse Stanley. How about if she asks Dr. Marquez to change his plan and give you something for pain. Will you try getting the X-rays then?"

Ms. Hellman: "I don't know. I don't think I could stand the pain of the needle."

Nurse Frost: "What needle?"

Ms. Hellman: "The one she said they're going to put into my kidney to make it light up."

Nurse Frost: "I think we've confused you."

Nurse Stanley: "I didn't mean that the needle would go into your kidney. The needle goes into your arm, like an IV or when they draw blood. The doctor then injects some fluid through the needle in your arm and the fluid will travel through your bloodstream and into your kidneys. After the tiny needle stick in your arm, you won't feel anything. No wonder you didn't want to get those X-rays."

Example #9 illustrates one type of conflict—a nursing professional who is unable to gain patient compliance. In spite of

Nurse Stanley's efforts to use reward power to persuade the patient, she was unsuccessful. Nurse Frost was able to determine the source of the conflict by listening to both interactants and by giving the patient an opportunity to communicate her anxiety. Frequently conflicts occur through miscommunication, such as the one shown in Example #9. Conflict resolution requires that you try to determine the reason for the conflict, rather than continuing to participate in a adult-child type of dialogue with lots of "either or" and "you can't make me" issues. Part of your role is to aid patients, their families, your peers, and other members of the health care team with conflict resolution. Your ability to open the channels of communication between the individuals involved in the conflict will determine how successful you and, ultimately, they will be. Try not to take sides in the discussion, but, rather, attempt to listen to both sides of the debate and encourage all interactants to discuss the basis for the conflict rather than fueling the conflict with idle threats and innuendo.

A great deal has been written about communicating with dying patients. Kubler-Ross (1969), among others, has discussed at great length the need to allow dying patients to express their feelings and concerns. This textbook is not intended to explore in-depth this important area of health communication. However, we would like to make a few key points.

1. If patients ask you questions about their illness, to the extent that you feel comfortable answering their questions, attempt to do so. If you feel that a doctor, a minister, or a relative should be discussing something the patient is concerned about, let the patient know your feelings and then advise the proper individual that the patient has some concerns and questions for him or her.

2. If the patient knows he or she is dying, don't try and negate the facts. You certainly do not have to be overly pessimistic or cynical about it, but if the patient is trying to accept the reality of his or her condition, do your best to help him or her, but don't sugarcoat it.

3. Encourage the family members to talk with the patient and vice versa. Sometimes patients want to talk with their relatives about their condition, but the family doesn't feel comfortable doing so.

Perhaps you can help both the relatives and the patients bridge the communication gap.

4. Finally, try to approach a dying patient as you would any other patient with a serious illness. If you were in the patient's place, you would want people to treat you with dignity and respect. Avoid the temptation to be overly optimistic or to ignore the patient because you don't want to discuss his or her impending death. Your ability to communicate as a caring, compassionate human being may be the best medicine anyone can provide to a patient in such a circumstance. Try to always approach communicating with dying patients, or any patient for that matter, with the golden rule—"How would I want a nursing professional to treat me and talk with me if I were in that position?" Most of us would choose a nursing professional who is empathetic, sincere, and compassionate. These qualities are easily demonstrated in your verbal and nonverbal communication with a dying patient.

INTERPERSONAL COMMUNICATION

In addition to your role as a communicator with patients, you will also be expected to communicate with a variety of other audiences: patients' families, physicians, nurses, and other health care professionals. This task is sometimes complicated by the hierarchical nature of health care, by the need for confidentiality, and by the multiple audiences, purposes, and uses for the information you possess about a patient.

Let's take a look at one example of a nurse-patient's family interaction. Try to assume the role of the nurse in this example, and ask yourself the question, "How could I communicate with these people more effectively, more clearly, and still demonstrate my professional competency and credibility?"

Example #10

Setting: A patient's home, the home health nurse has just arrived for her daily visit with Mrs. Lexington, a terminally ill cancer patient who is receiving morphine via an intravenous pump. The patient is doing much worse than the day before, and, after the nurse assesses the patient, she is confronted by the family.

Nurse Simms: "Mrs. Lexington must have had a rough night."

Mr. Lexington: "We thought we were going to lose her."

Nurse Simms: "You know, she's only going to get worse. You can't expect too much. I'll be by again tomorrow, and if you have any questions, call me."

Fay Lexington: "We think mom should be in the hospital."

Nurse Simms: "Who's we?"

Tom Lexington: "Dad, Fay, and I. We just don't know what to do for her."

Nurse Simms: "Look, we've been through all this. Doctor Alonzo told you that there's nothing else to do for her. So, all we can do is make her comfortable. Now I'll be back tomorrow."

Here is an all too typical example of a problem that home health nurses face almost daily. A terminal patient becomes gradually more incapacitated and the family, even though they intellectually realize that nothing else can be done, want to have all possible avenues of help available. If it was your parent or significant other and you didn't have your health care training and experience, you might feel the same way. They don't want to look back after mom's dead and wonder if they could've done something that would have extended their time together. It may not be realistic, but guilt and anxiety are not usually founded on realism.

Please answer the following questions about Example #10:

1. Did the nurse explain the changes in the patient's condition to the family and what they could expect to happen next?

   yes _____   unsure_____   no _____

2. Did the nurse explain to the family why the patient would not benefit from being hospitalized?

   yes _____   unsure _____   no _____

3. Did you perceive this nurse as being compassionate and empathic with the family's ordeal?

   yes _____   unsure _____   no _____

4. List as many reasons as you can to explain why the family wanted to move mom to the hospital.

In order to determine some of these answers, let's revise the conversation of Example #10 and let the family and the nurse discover them for us.

Example #11

Nurse Simms: "Mrs. Lexington must've had a rough night."

Mr. Lexington: "We thought we were going to lose her."

Nurse Simms: "It must be very difficult for you. I understand that it isn't easy to watch someone you love die."

Fay Lexington: "No, it's not, that's why we think mom should be in the hospital."

Nurse Simms: "Well, let's talk about that. Why do you feel that way?"

Tom Lexington: "We're scared. We don't know what to do for her and we don't want her to die if they could do something for her."

Nurse Simms: "I understand how you feel. When I first started as a home health nurse, I felt the same way. I mean there's something very safe about all the people working in a hospital with all that equipment and all the machines. But you know what I finally learned?"

Fay Lexington: "What?"

Nurse Simms: "I learned that the hospital's a great place to be if you need treatment and you've got a chance to get well. But if you're so ill that there aren't any machines or any medicine that will make you better and you can be just as comfortable at home—with the people who love you—most of us want to be at home. So I'll bet if you think about it, you'll realize that your mom would rather be here. She's got oxygen and morphine, and that's all they could do for her in the hospital, but, most importantly, this is where she spent her life, with you. I'm sure from the little while I've known her that she'd much rather be here with her things and the people who love her than in a sterile, strange hospital. Now, I'll be glad to call Doctor Alonzo, tell him about your concerns, and see if he wants to put Mrs. Lexington back into the hospital, if that's what you want?"

Mr. Lexington: "No, you're right. We're just afraid, and we don't want to lose her."

Nurse Simms: "I know, and if there was anything else that could be done Doctor Alonzo would have put her in the hospital. But now that we know we can't cure her illness, maybe we can be less afraid and just try to comfort her and make her as pain-free as possible."

Tom Lexington: "Thanks, I think we just needed someone to explain it to us again. It's hard to watch your mom die."

Nurse Simms: "I know it is, and that's why I'm here—to help as much as I can. Please, next time you get concerned, call. If I'm not on call, one of the other nurses will answer your questions or come out and check on her. Let me just mention that I think her breathing is going to gradually get more and more difficult. She'll probably start gasping for air occasionally, and she may even have some periods of time when she isn't breathing. That's the way this disease effects the brain. So, maybe it will help for you to know that as the pressure on her brain increases from the tumor, she's going to be more and more unresponsive, in a coma, and gradually her breathing will become more affected."

Fay Lexington: "Thanks, at least we'll know what to expect. It gets pretty scary when you don't know what's going on."

Nurse Simms: "I know. Now please call if you need me and remember, you're doing everything you can for her."

The family in Example #11, when given the opportunity, is more than willing to share their concerns, questions, and fears. In Example #11 Nurse Simms is both a listener and a responder. She is compassionate, empathic, informative, supportive, and willing to follow the family's wishes. This approach, instead of the "I'm the medical authority here and I know what's right" approach, empowers the family by providing them with information and options. In this example everyone is more satisfied with the communication exchange because it is a dyadic exchange and not an authoritarian blitzkrieg.

A major problem with authoritarian interactions is that they do not allow the interactants to exchange information. Instead, the authoritarian-interactant often precludes any exchange by turning a dialogue into a monologue. This type of interaction can occur in a variety of contexts. One such context was illustrated in Example #10. Another example can be shown in a nurse-physician interaction.

Example #12

Setting: The nurse's desk in a large hospital. Nurse Jackson is talking on the telephone to Doctor Bowers about his patient, Mr. Lumbata, who has been complaining about abdominal pain.

Nurse Jackson: "Hello, Dr. Bowers, this is Canera Jackson, I'm on three-West at County General and I'm concerned about your patient Mr. Lumbata in Room 373. He's called me down to his room twice in the past half-hour to complain about his abdomen hurting. He says it's the worst pain he's ever felt."

Dr. Bowers: "Isn't he the patient that was admitted with chest pain and anxiety?"

Nurse Jackson: "Yes, but . . ."

Dr. Bowers: "Well, I wouldn't get too worked up about his complaints. He's probably just anxious again. Give him five milligrams of Valium p.o. and see if that doesn't fix his bellyache."

Nurse Jackson: "O.K., but, . . ."

This conversation is not atypical of many interactions that occur in medicine. Countless nurses have experienced similar situations to the one depicted in Example #12. You hang up the phone after being cut off by a physician, concerned that you have not represented the best interests of the patient, but acutely aware of the hierarchical nature of the medical world. In Example #12 Doctor Bowers uses his expert power (see Chapter 2) to inform Nurse Jackson of what should be done for the patient. Nurse Jackson is ineffective in utilizing her legitimate power (see Chapter 2) to communicate her concerns and the reasons for her apprehension. In the space below rewrite Example #12 and try to use language choices that are more assertive and persuasive.

As we discussed in chapters 2 and 3, competent communication requires communication behaviors that are appropriate for the situation. Obviously, in Example #12 a physician does not believe, based on the information she or he received, that the nurse's concerns about a patient's complaints merit further evaluation. Therefore, a quick-fix prescription for Valium is verbally ordered for the anxious patient and nonverbally for the benefit of the concerned nurse. ("Maybe that'll satisfy her and she'll leave me alone.") The problem for readers of this example, and all too frequently for jurors in a courtroom where these kinds of interactions are recanted, is that the nurse's tone, the fact that she calls the doctor, intimates that she is concerned based on her assessment of the patient's complaints.

Readers of Example #12 know that the nurse has seen the patient more recently than the physician, and that the nurse has the advantage of having communicated with the patient both before, during, and after his complaints of abdominal pain. Thus, it is the nurse's responsibility to communicate precisely and persuasively information about the patient that Dr. Bowers needs to determine an effective course of action. After Dr. Bowers tried to dismiss the patient's complaint by reminding the nurse of the patient's diagnosis of anxiety, the nurse could have used objective data to support the legitimacy of the patient's complaints.

Example #13

For example, Nurse Jackson might have said, "Yes doctor, he did present with anxiety and chest pain. On admission, however, the patient was afebrile, but he now has a temperature of 102.5 degrees and his pulse, which was normal an hour ago, is now 124. His blood pressure has dropped from normal range to 104 over 60, and his color is pale and he's diaphoretic. I couldn't hear any bowel sounds when I listened for a full minute, and his abdomen, which was soft earlier, is now hard and painful to the touch. It wasn't that way when my shift started four hours ago."

This description is much more informative and persuasive. It provides both the nurse and the doctor a chance to interact further, and it relies on objective data in addition to the patient's and the nurse's subjective statements about the pain. Such a statement might have caused Doctor Bowers to ask, "Did he eat his supper?" This question would have given Nurse Jackson an opportunity to provide more detailed information about the patient's anorexia and nausea. While it is true that Doctor Bowers is ultimately responsible for the patient's medical care, Nurse Jackson is responsible for the patient's nursing care and for making certain that Doctor Bowers is well-informed and equipped with enough subjective and objective data to assess the patient's condition and determine a course of action or treatment. On occasion, you may even need to call a physician a second time and restate your concerns and assessment in order to assure that he or she understood what you were attempting to communicate. Finally, as we will discuss in Chapter 6, this is exactly the kind of information (the patient's complaint, your assessment of the objective data, your communication of that information to the physician, and the physician's response) that you should carefully record and communicate in the medical record.

It should be pointed out that nurse-physician interactions are by no means the only contexts influenced by hierarchy. In addition to settings such as the one described in Example #12, there are also countless encounters between nurses and their supervisors. These hierarchical interactions can have either a satisfactory or an unsatisfactory result based solely on the willingness of the two interactants to exchange information as adults, rather than one interactant choosing to make demands and use the opportunity to provide a monologue, instead of engaging in dyadic communication.

Examples #14 and #15 are typical conversations between a nurse and a nursing supervisor. Try to determine if these are primarily monologues governed by an authoritarian "dictator," or a dialogue between two nursing professionals, one of whom is a supervisor.

Example #14

Setting: A nurses' station. Nursing Supervisor Yancey is talking to Nurse Atmore. The supervisor is loud and pointing a finger at the younger, obviously intimidated nurse.

Supervisor Yancey: "Did you forget to chart some information on any patients last night?"

Nurse Atmore: "I don't think so, but maybe. It was after midnight before we finished the code, and I knew I wasn't supposed to be on overtime. I tried to get my charting done as quickly as I could, I guess I could've forgotten something."

Supervisor Yancey: "Well, your rushing to get done nearly cost the patient in 622 his life. You didn't chart that the patient had fallen on your shift. During the night he became confused and had seizures. Luckily, Dr. Winston saw a bruise on the back of his head and ordered a CT scan. He had a subdural hematoma and had to have burr holes. He's better today, but no thanks to you."

Compare Example #14 with the following interaction:

Example #15

Setting: Supervisor's office. Supervisor Albertti is seated opposite nurse Patrick.

Supervisor Albertti: "I heard there were some problems last night with Mr. Tompkins. What exactly happened?"

Nurse Patrick: "Well, one of the new R.N.s did Mr. Tompkin's fingerstick at bedtime and it was low, so she gave him some orange juice before she notified Dr. Miller about the results."

Supervisor Albertti: "What did Dr. Miller have to say?"

Nurse Patrick: "He wanted to know why he wasn't notified first, since he wanted to get a glucose level drawn before the patient got any juice. The nurse reminded him that his standing orders called for treatment with orange juice and sugar in patients who are alert and then notification of the physician."

Supervisor Albertti: "Did that satisfy him?"

Nurse Patrick: "I'm not sure anything satisfies Dr. Miller, but I think it calmed him down. Helen, it was her patient, she and I discussed it later and she agreed that in the future she'll call the doctor while someone else gets the orange juice ready. That way she can avoid being placed in a difficult spot."

Supervisor Albertti: "That sounds like a good solution. She complies with the protocol and attempts to accommodate Dr. Miller's request to be notified at the same time. I think I'll draft a memo to the staff suggesting that they do the same thing in similar situations. Plus, I'll tell Dr. Miller so he's aware of our efforts to meet both his patient's needs and his changing protocol."

Please answer the following questions about Examples #14 and #15.

1. Are either or both of these supervisors communicating effectively with the nurses?

   yes _____   unsure _____   no _____

   If so, why and how? _____

   _____

2. If you had to discuss a problem with a nursing supervisor who responded like one of the supervisors in these two examples, which supervisor's communication style would you choose for your supervisor and why?

   _____

   _____

   _____

One of the lessons to be gained from these two examples is that learning can be influenced either positively or negatively. In Example #14, Nurse Atmore has been educated about future charting; however, her feelings about this interaction and the way in which she was instructed are most likely going to be extremely negative. On the other hand, Nurse Patrick not only receives positive feedback from her supervisor, but she also appears to have engaged in an effective form of communication with the new nurse who had the problem with Doctor Miller. The key to Example #15 is that the nursing professionals did not accept this incident as merely "Doctor Miller's picking on us again" (which she or he may have been doing), nor did they scoff at the physician for not recalling his or her own protocol.

Instead, the nurses found a means to improve their future communication with each other, Doctor Miller, and still treat the patient. In this way, everyone—the nursing staff, Doctor Miller, and most of all the patient—benefits. That is obviously the goal of effective health communication, and Example #15 illustrates it for us.

Let's see if you can rewrite Example #14 in the space below and make it a more effective, positive, communication experience for both of the interactants. Keep in mind that accurate and thorough charting needed to be done before the nurse went home, but the verbal and nonverbal communication of that information could be much more compassionate and persuasive.

By now, you probably have surmised that one of the nonverbal elements of Example #14 that immediately signals a problem is the setting for this highly charged interaction. Just as we don't teach college classes in a parking lot (too many distractions and a poor environment for learning), we don't critique professionals in front of their peers and others (too disconfirming and unnecessarily humiliating). Supervisor Yancey can set a totally different tone for this interaction by calmly asking Nurse Atmore to come by the supervisor's office. Other nonverbal behaviors that are frequently perceived as dictatorial and generally humiliating are: pointing an "accusing" finger at someone, a harsh tone of voice, and the use of sarcasm.

Example #16

Having discussed the role of nonverbal behavior in disconfirming interactions, let's revisit the two interactants, but this time in Supervisor Yancey's office. The two professionals are seated a few feet from each other, and Supervisor Yancey is speaking in a soft voice, being careful to maintain eye contact with Nurse Atmore.

Supervisor Yancey: "Monica, what can you tell me about your patient, Mr. Gleason. Did something happen to him last night before you left?"

Nurse Atmore: "I feel just awful. He fell just as I was getting ready to leave. I told Sally, but I was running late, and with the new policy about overtime, I rushed my charting and forgot to chart that he fell. I heard about his surgery, and I feel just awful about it."

Supervisor Yancey: "I know, and I'm sure it wasn't your fault he fell; I heard he climbed over the rails. I'm not trying to blame someone, I'm just trying to determine what happened and see if we can't come up with a solution that will prevent a similar incident from happening again. It just so happened that Sally's daughter got very ill and Sally had to leave about 30 minutes after you did, so no one knew anything about Mr. Gleason's fall. We really do put you new nurses in a bind by trying to keep costs down and discouraging overtime and yet expecting you to make sure that all your work is done before you go."

Nurse Atmore: "It's really hard to get everything done, remember all my charting, and still leave on time."

Supervisor Yancey: "I realize that and I know you did the best you could given the situation. You've made a good point. I think we'll try to get some seminars on charting, but we also need to work on clarifying our policy so no one gets stuck in the uncomfortable and potentially dangerous position you were in. What do you think we could do to make the policy clearer and easier to follow?"

In addition to interacting with supervisors, nursing professionals communicate with countless other members of the health care team, many of whom see themselves as subordinate to the nurse in terms of the medical hierarchy. You will find other health care professionals much more willing to assist you and cooperate in the care of patients if you allow them to take part in the decision-making process as much as possible. Treat them as professionals, communicate with, not at, them, and you will find effective communication much easier to achieve. Successful interactions, from a communication perspective, can take place in any context, (e.g., supervisors, peers, or subordinates) if the interactants allow information to be exchanged rather than dictated, and if power is mutually achieved instead of unilaterally invoked.

We have discussed a number of verbal and nonverbal settings for communication; however, professional nurses also are responsible for the intricacies of written communication, as well.

5

Communicating in
the Medical Record

In freshman composition class you were taught that writing is
a process (Scholes & Comley, 1981; Troyka, 1987). Like verbal
and nonverbal communication, written communication is not
a linear operation. Instead, an author uses a process to communicate in writing. This process involves the continual back and
forth nature of analyzing, informing, reassessing, and review-
ing/revising what is being communicated. This process of writing can be divided into three separate, but interdependent
stages: prewriting, writing, and reviewing (Scholes & Comley,
1981; Troyka, 1987).

Professional nurses create a wide variety of written documents, from memos and letters to admission assessments and
Nurses Notes. In addition, Community and Home Health nurses
author various other documents and Emergency Room, Obstetrics, and Operating Room nurses create still different sets of
records. This text will discuss many of these records; however,
we will not deal with letters or memos, nor will we discuss
Nursing Care Plans. Because of the recent deletion by the Joint
Commission on Accreditation of Healthcare Organizations
(JCAHO) of a standard for Nursing Care Plans in hospitals, we

will not evaluate their usefulness. James Parsek, R.N. (1991), the Associate Director of the JCAHO Department of Standards states, "Did the Joint Commission eliminate care plans? Yes! [There is no reference in the AMH/91 [Accreditation Manual for Hospitals] (or the 1992 edition) to any requirement for a care plan" (p. 2).]

PREWRITING

To analyze the information needed in a written document, an author must determine the audience who is most likely to read it (Mathis & Stevenson, 1980; Mills & Walter, 1978). Consequently, nurse-authors must determine who the primary and secondary readers are for any medical record they write. In addition, you need to understand the many purposes for authoring a medical record and determine how you as a writer want readers to use the document.

Let's look at an example of prewriting analyses. While you are in nursing school, you are assigned to write Nurses Notes on your care and evaluation of a patient. Your primary audience in that instance will be your professor, and the secondary audience will be your classmates. Some of the purposes for writing this medical record for your professor include the need to demonstrate your mastery of patient interview skills, physical examination techniques, your ability to assess a patient's illness, her or his responses to the illness, and your competency at communicating your assessment, nursing diagnosis, and interventions in a medical record. In addition, you want your professor to use the document to improve your grade and allow you to progress further in your nursing education.

You should also realize that your peers are a secondary audience for this document, and they have a different use for the record—they want to learn from your communication successes and failures. Your peers want to determine, from your example, how to effectively communicate information about a patient to the professor and other readers. You want your colleagues to use the record as a stellar model of properly authored Nurses

Notes and thus an example of your evolving competency and burgeoning credibility as a professional nurse.

The potential audiences for any document are determined by the purpose and use of the record. For example, the primary audience for Nurses Notes in a hospital setting include: your peers, who will also be caring for the patient; the patient's physician and any consultants; and other members of the health care team who may need information about the patient in order to carry out their duties (e.g., a respiratory therapy technician may use the record to determine if a patient has experienced any breathing difficulties since his or her last treatment). There are also numerous secondary audiences for these records. The secondary audiences include administrators, nursing supervisors, quality assurance and peer reviewers, researchers, nursing students, and malpractice attorneys. While it is true that the secondary audience's use of the medical record may not have a direct effect on the patient's care and treatment, this audience's use of the record is still vitally important to the nurse-author's purpose for writing the document. For example, many Nursing Directors use Nurses Notes as a major tool in determining their staff's performance for yearly raises. Thus the medical record you create is frequently used to determine the level of expertise you have, your professional competency, and how well you communicate those attributes to others. Attorney Walter Killian (1991) writes,

Although the primary purposes of the medical record are to provide a complete and accurate documentary of the care and treatment a patient receives while in the hospital, and to provide a means of communication between all members of the treatment team, the medical record serves another important purpose. As the chronicle of the patient's treatment in the hospital, it may someday be used as evidence in a law suit brought by a patient alleging negligent treatment. (p. 22)

The simple one- or two-page record that you author to describe your evaluation of the patient and her or his response to treatment is being used by numerous individuals for countless purposes. Your task as the author of such a multifarious document is to be certain that it communicates effectively and persuasively to the multiple audiences who use it.

We discussed in chapters 1, 2, and 3 the importance of demonstrating your credibility and competency in order to persuade an audience. Nowhere is the need for such demonstration more important than in a medical record. Killian (1991) supports this belief when he states, "To a large extent, the care with which the documentation was kept will reflect on the quality of care the patient received, such that if a nurse's documentation is sloppy, incomplete, or inaccurate, the jury may well conclude that the nurse provided care to patients in much the same way" (p. 22).

Let's look at the following verbatim transcription of an anonymous patient's Nurses Notes and answer the questions that follow the document. Try to determine how the communication in the record might affect your opinion of the nurse-author's competency and/or credibility.

Record #1

Nurses Notes

7:40 p.m.: 70 yr. old female admitted to room 208A via amb.
8:15 p.m.: Settled in room. States does not want sleeping pill.
9:25 p.m.: To X-ray via w/c.
10:00 p.m.: Good 3 hours.

Please answer the following questions about Record #1

1. What is the reason for the patient's hospitalization?

_____

2. What do you think is meant by "Settled in room"?

_____

3. Why would the nurse be discussing a sleeping pill if the patient is scheduled to go for an X-ray 45 minutes later?

4. If your answer to Question #3 was that the x-ray was unscheduled, what type of X-ray was ordered and why was it suddenly ordered after nine o'clock at night?

5. According to the Nurses Notes, the patient has only been in her room 2 hours and 20 minutes, therefore, which statement in Record #1 is incorrect—the admission and final record times of 7:40 and 10:00 or the "Good 3 hours"?

If you had difficulty answering any or all of these questions, you are beginning to understand the problems readers of medical records face. This very brief and noninformative note is typical of many of the Nurses Notes we reviewed. The use of short, cryptic, nonsentences to communicate information does little except confuse and frustrate a reader. Killian (1991) reinforces this belief when he writes, "The most important rule of good charting is that all entries in the medical record be complete, accurate, and timely. First there is the classic problem of undercharting. There is a well established maxim stating that if something isn't documented, it didn't occur" (p. 22). Even more alarming than the confusion such writing creates is the lack of persuasion this type of noncommunication evokes. Ask yourself, would I trust my mother to a nurse who writes such confusing notes? Can you feel confident, based on this record, that the nurse is not just as careless in her assessments and delivery of medication as she or he is in her or his documentation?

The important lessons in this example are: your professional credibility and competency frequently are evaluated by readers who have nothing else to use in assessing your work, except your documentation in the Nurses Notes; readers, who only have access to the written record, must be persuaded that the nurse's assessments, nursing diagnoses, and interventions were meticulously performed, accurately accomplished, and intelligently derived. When a nurse-author is scrupulous in his or her written communication, an audience can be persuaded that the nurse is competent and credible and that his or her actions and opinions are grounded in sound nursing theory.

The purpose for Nurses Notes then, is not unidimensional but, rather, multidimensional. Like most written communication, you create Nurses Notes to inform *and* persuade readers. Your task, however, is onerous indeed, because you are attempting to provide scientific information to a vast audience and at the same time demonstrate your professional competency and credibility and avoid any hint of malpractice or malfeasance. You want your diverse audiences to use the medical record to learn about the patient's evolving medical condition, the course of her or his treatment, your current assessment, nursing diagnoses, and the results of your interventions.

Armed with the knowledge that your audience is diverse, your purposes in creating Nurses Notes are multidimensional, and the use of the documents are varied, you are now ready to proceed to the next stage in the writing process and actually begin to put words on paper. Remember, however, that since writing is a process, you will be continually assessing and reassessing your writing against your prewriting analyses of the audience, purpose, and use for the record to assure that the document communicates effectively for its intended audience, purpose, and use.

WRITING

To effectively communicate information in writing, an author must know the appropriate format and style for the type of document being authored. Thus an author who writes a novel in the format and style of an essay will find it extremely difficult to convince an audience that he or she knows anything about writing a novel. When an informed and experienced audience's expectations are not met, the author's competency and credibility are called into question.

Countless readers of medical records expect the documents to follow the accepted formats prescribed in the Joint Commission on Accreditation of Healthcare Organizations' guidelines. The 1991 JCAHO *Accreditation Manual for Hospitals* lists the following requirements:

> NC.1.3.4 The patient's medical record includes documentation of
>
> NC.1.3.4.1 The initial assessments and reassessments;
>
> NC.1.3.4.2 The nursing diagnoses and/or patient care needs;
>
> NC.1.3.4.3 The interventions identified to meet the patient's nursing care needs;
>
> NC.1.3.4.4 The nursing care provided;
>
> NC.1.3.4.5 The patient's response to, and the outcomes of, the care provided; and
>
> NC.1.3.4.6 The ability of the patient and/or, as appropriate, his/her significant other(s) to manage continuing care needs after discharge. (p. 132)

The only way for a nurse-author to communicate the detailed information required by JCAHO is to provide clear and sufficient data in a standardized format that meets an audience's expectations and needs. Nurse Parsek (1991), of the JCAHO, states, "When problems with nursing documentation surface during a Joint Commission survey, usually it is not the mechanism, as such, but the fact that nursing care is not being documented that causes surveyors to recommend changes" (p. 2). Clearly, nurse-writers can persuade readers and JCAHO surveyors by supplying information that was properly and scientifically obtained, carefully analyzed, meticulously described, and accurately reported.

PERSUASION

Persuasion and the effective communication of information rely on an author's language choices, demonstration of professionalism, and careful assessment of the data being presented.

Therefore, *a nurse-author can communicate more effectively and persuasively if she or he uses language that is appropriate for the audience, descriptive, clear, and concise.* A nurse-writer demonstrates his or her professionalism through the use of a proper format and an acceptable writing style. In order for a reader to evaluate the writer's assessments and actions, an author needs to make language choices that clearly inform readers and explain any ambiguities. Finally, the nurse-author needs to clarify any obtuse aspects of his or her assessment of a patient's illness or treatment. An audience cannot be expected to reach the same hypotheses as an author, unless the author provides all the details and information necessary to allow readers to arrive at the same conclusions as the nurse-author.

In order for a reader to derive similar conclusions and nursing diagnoses, nurse-writers should remember that readers need to be able to follow the author's logic and deduction. Scattered bits of information or a declaration from the nurse as to the meaning of the information, in place of the actual data, does not allow an audience to assimilate important findings and results in order to reach the same conclusions/diagnoses as the nurse-author. Killian (1991) emphatically states, "Be factual and specific, and avoid generalizations. In terms of the information provided to other health care workers and the defensibility of the record there is a big difference between the statement, 'The patient is doing fine,' and a systems assessment focusing on the patient's injured system" (p. 22). It is critical for nurse-authors to remember that persuasion results from the effective communication of information, not the mere recording of subjective statements or innuendo.

In recent years some nursing departments have turned to flow sheets in an attempt to ease the paperwork burden on their nursing staff. However, this seemingly inconsequential shift from clearly stated information to "objectively" reported "facts," is far from irrelevant. Evaluate Record #2 (Figure 5.1), an 8-hour shift of a 24-hour flow sheet, obtained from a JCAHO-accredited hospital, and be prepared to answer questions about it. Try to ascertain from the flow sheet how a reader can assess changes in a patient's condition over an 8-hour period and how

ASSESSMENT: 2300 - 0700

DATE/TIME 5/5/91

Nurse Signature

NEUROLOGICAL

LOC: Alert to— person		☑ Yes	☐ No
place		☑ Yes	☐ No
time		☑ Yes	☐ No
Speech clear		☑ Yes	☐ No
Presence of pain		☑ Yes	☐ No
Hand grip equal		☑ Yes	☐ No
Moves all extremities		☑ Yes	☐ No

SKIN

☑ warm	☑ dry	☐ pink	☐ brown	☐ black
☐ pale	☐ moist	☐ flushed	☐ diaphoretic	
☐ clammy	☐ dusky	☐ cool	☐ cyanotic	
☐ jaundice	☐ other_____			
Turgor		☐ normal	☐ abnormal	

CARDIOVASCULAR

Peripheral pulses equal		☑ Yes	☐ No
Capillary Refill	☑ immediate	☐ prolonged	

IV/HL Site:

☑ clear	☐ redness	☐ swelling	☐ drainage

☐ warm to touch

Sol. Rate/# _____ LR Ⓐ 75ᶜᶜ/HR _____

Edema:	Extremities	☐ Yes	☑ No
	Sacral	☐ Yes	☑ No
	Periorbital	☐ Yes	☐ No
Pain with dorsiflexion:	Right	☐ Yes	☑ No
	Left	☐ Yes	☑ No
Heart sounds normal		☑ Yes	☐ No

Telemetry rhythm _____

Fig. 5.1. 8-Hour Shift of a 24–Hour Nursing Flow Sheet

94

RESPIRATORY

Rate normal   ☑ Yes   ☐ No

Lung sounds

☐ clear ☑ raies ☐ rhonchi ☐ wheezes ☐ labored

☐ SOB ☐ retraction   ☐ decreased ☐ absent

Cough productive   ☑ Yes   ☐ No

☐ Chest tubes

GASTROINTESTINAL

Bowel sounds in all 4 quadrants

☑ active ☐ hypoactive   ☐ hyperactive ☐ absent

Abdomen ☐ soft   ☐ distended ☐ tender

Presence of ☐ vomiting   ☐ diarrhea   ☐ nausea

Ostomy site_____

☐ NG   ☐ Hi   ☐ Lo

Other_____

GENITOURINARY

Urine color ☑ amber   ☐ dark amber

☐ pale   ☐ concentrated ☐ other

Tubes   ☐ foley   ☐ aupropubic

Bladder distended   ☐ Yes   ☐ No

Other_____

MUSCULOSKELETAL

Normal   ☑ Yes   ☐ No

Mobility ☐ turns self   ☑ needs help

Other_____

SURGICAL INCISION/WOUNDS

Site   ☐ clean ☐ dry ☐ pink ☐ red

Dressing ☐ dry   ☐ clean ☐ soiled ☐ wet

Drainage ☐ none ☐ scant ☐ small

    ☐ medium ☐ large

 color _brown_____

 odor ☐ absent ☐ present

Drains_____

_____ penrose _____

Other_____

*All abnormals to be charted on the Nurses Notes.

Fig. 5.1. Continued

a nurse can use such a form to describe any alterations that occur during his or her 8 hours with a patient?

Record #2

Nursing Flow Sheet Questionnaire

1. How would you know, based on this flow sheet, if a patient's assessment was made before or after an unexpected event?

   _____

2. The asterisk at the bottom of the page states, "All abnormals to be charted on the Nurses Notes." What, then, is the purpose of this flow sheet?

   _____

3. How many different medical conditions can you think of that would require hospitalization and yet have no abnormal assessments?

   _____

The problem with flow sheets, as illustrated by the example in Record #2, are not that they simply record data, but that they document only data that fits the specific flow sheet format. You must be able to check a preprinted box, in order to supply information on the flow sheet. But ask yourself the question, if all that is necessary for patient care is a simple yes or no response to a series of questions on a page, then why do nurses need a college degree and continuing education? After all, a computer and an automatic blood pressure machine could supply most of the information requested on the flow sheet in Record #2. However, the value of highly educated and skilled nurses is their ability to translate data into assessments, nursing diagnoses, and interventions. Therefore, the simple checklist system generally does not decrease the work load for nurses, but instead, it frequently serves to increase it. The extra work comes from the fact that the nondescriptive check marks must be translated into meaningful communication about the assessment, nursing diagnosis, interventions, and the results of those interventions. In the space that follows, please write a Nurses Note that restates the information supplied by the flow sheet in Record #2.

Let's now look at a possible example that uses objective data from the flow sheet to describe an 8-hour assessment of a fictional patient. Since many nursing and legal authorities suggest that Nurses Notes be written frequently and some even require that notes be recorded every two hours. Killian (1991) reminds nurses that,

> It is important that entries in the medical record be made as close in time to the observation or the service provided as possible. This will serve several purposes. First, it ensures that the information is available for other health care professionals involved in the treatment of the patient. Second, it helps ensure that the information that is recorded is as accurate, complete, and reliable as possible. (p. 22)

Record #3

Nurses Notes—Example #1

2300:   Ms. Jones is asleep, breathing without difficulty. She arouses easily and is oriented to time, place, and person. Her vital signs are normal and her IV is infusing at 75 cc/hr. Her breath sounds are improved over yesterday, but there are occasional crackles in the left lung. She is not on oxygen, her nails are pink and her capillary refill is brisk. Her penrose has a scant amount of brownish discharge.

0100:   Ms. Jones' piggyback of Ancef 1 gm. is started and infusing without difficulty. She is still oriented x 3, PERRLA, her speech is clear and her grip strength is equal in both hands.

0300:   The patient is sleeping and awakens just long enough to answer questions. She remains oriented x 3 and her IV site in her left anterior forearm is not reddened or swollen. She is off oxygen and without any respiratory distress.

0500:   Ms. Jones continues to be oriented x 3. She has normal active bowel sounds, and a nontender abdomen. Ms. Jones denies any pain, "I feel much better than I did when I came here three days ago."

0700:   Ms. Jones had a quiet night, remains alert, oriented to time, place, and person and "hungry this morning." Her rales persist in the left base, but without rhonchi or wheezes and she denies any shortness of breath. She had 265 ccs of urinary output and 600 ccs of IV intake.

In less space than is occupied by a flow sheet, this record provides a reader with detailed and descriptive information about a nurse's encounters, assessments, and treatment of this patient. Any abnormal findings are discussed when they are noted, and the reader does not have to look elsewhere to discover information about the patient's neuro checks, vital signs, IV, intake and output, antibiotics, and assessment. The clarity and informative nature of this brief note, when compared to the flow sheet, are obvious. This note provides the same data, but allows the nurse-author to describe any changes in the patient's condition over the past 8 hours. This note makes it clear to a reader what events occurred during the shift, the quantity of the patient's intake and output, and the patient's own statement about her condition. It is true that a reader could have discovered most of this information by reading the check marks on the flow sheet, but the reader would then have to go to a separate page for an explanation of the abnormal lung sounds, a different page for the patient's intake and output, and a third page for the patient's antibiotic administration.

In Chapter 6 we will discuss some specific methods you can use to document your patient's condition, nursing diagnosis, and interventions. You can see from this brief discussion about using a flow sheet versus a well-written chronology that simply recording objective data does not communicate clearly and concisely what you see and assess about your patient's illness, treatment, and recovery. Your role as a nurse-author is to communicate more than mere check marks. Your role is to inform readers about the patient's condition and to persuade an audience that the quality of your assessment and care is above reproach.

REVIEWING

One of the aspects of medical-record writing that is frequently overlooked is the reviewing or editing stage of the process. In this day and age when so many medical records are being dictated, transcribed, and later signed by authors, the potential for mistakes is compounded by the number of people involved in creating the final text and the amount of time dedicated to authoring and reviewing it.

Let's digress for just a moment to add our personal feelings to the debate about dictated versus handwritten Nurses Notes. We firmly believe that a dictated or word-processed, transcribed, and typed/printed medical record is the medically and legally safest, clearest, and most effective form of written communication. We say this because handwritten documents suffer due to countless problems with legibility. You may have the most readable handwriting in the world, but if you do you are in a minority. Most of us struggle to make our handwriting legible for ourselves, let alone for numerous readers who are unaccustomed to our egocentric penmanship styles. Furthermore, you may be able to read your scribble today, minutes after you write it, but what about two or three years from now when you are seated in a court room and the attorney asks you to swear that you can clearly read the document.

It is true that typed records have their shortcomings as well. Frequently there are delays in getting the transcription on a patient's chart in a timely manner, and too often there are typos and mistakes. But modern hospitals should be able to assign unit/ward clerks to type Nurses Notes or make arrangements with the Medical Records Department to have the Nurses Notes transcribed immediately after they are dictated. It will save you time, the hospital money, and it will likely help you both avoid the unnecessary stress of malpractice litigation. As for the mistakes and typos, part of your job as a writer is to review and revise the typed or written document prior to signing it, so you should catch any mistakes before they become a legal part of the record. Even more promising, however, is the newest trend toward computerized Nurses Notes. Hospitals that are experimenting with computers at the bedside or at the Nurses' Desk, provide nurses with secret passwords that they can use to access the patient's computerized record and create Nurses Notes for their patients. The password, which is usually changed biannually to assure confidentiality, is one mechanism to subvert the patients' and administrators' fears that anyone who has access to the hospital's computer could read or alter a patient's file. In addition, computerized medical records can be read by the patient's doctor, who has her or his own password, or the Nurses Notes can be printed out and placed in the chart at anytime. The advantages to computerized Nurses Notes are numerous, some of which include clarity, timeliness, neatness, and economics. Computerized Nurses Notes, when they are printed out, provide the clarity of typed notes. Plus they are usually more readily available than typed notes because the nurse-authors enter the notes into the computer themselves.

As we have already discussed, typed or computerized Nurses Notes are neater, and, therefore, easier to read; and, because no additional staff is needed to type the record, they are somewhat cost-effective. (The initial cost of the computers and printers can be offset by the savings in typists, or the legal ramifications associated with illegible handwritten notes.) The disadvantages, though few, continue to plague advocates of computerized medical records. Computers are expensive and, in addition to providing each Nurses' Desk with a computer and a printer, an institution needs a computer programmer available to maintain the software programs, as well as an electronics technician to maintain the computer hardware, and the hospital still has to purchase the necessary supplies for the equipment. As you can see, it is much more expensive to use a computerized system than a ballpoint pen or even an electric typewriter. In addition, if someone illicitly obtains your password, she or he has access to countless patients' confidential files, something that is greatly feared in this age of AIDS neurosis and insurance rejections. Perhaps even more frightening is the realization that anyone who has access to a computerized file can alter it without the original author of the document knowing about it.

One more important point about computerized records—the computer, in and of itself, *cannot* improve the basic aspects of written communication, prewriting, writing, and reviewing. Authors of computerized documents must still analyze their audience, use language choices and persuasion to meet that audience's needs and expectations, and review and revise the documents to achieve the effective written communication they desire.

The advantages to computerized medical records, especially the fact that Nurses Notes can be printed and on the chart before the nurse leaves the facility without the expense of a typist, makes this latest innovation extremely appealing. Plus, these printed records would be easier to review and correct prior to signing them; however, this point is also one of the legal drawbacks to computerized records. A person can edit a computerized document at *any time* without the computer demonstrating that a change has occurred (no white-out marks, eraser-smears, or crossed-out words). In other words, it would be difficult for you to prove that the Nurses Notes in Mr. X's chart were not altered (by you or someone else who has access to the computer's medical records) after the patient requested a copy of the record for his or her attorney. This issue of access is the biggest problem for authors of medical records, because unlike handwritten or typed Nurses Notes, you may have difficulty proving that the computer-generated record was not altered at a later time by you or someone else.

These are the advantages and disadvantages to computerized Nurses Notes. It would seem that the positive aspects would make them a valuable addition to every institution. We are confident that with time the disadvantages will be markedly reduced or eliminated and indeed it is probable that medical records of the not too distant future will all be computerized.

Remember—a document is not a legal part of the medical record *until you sign it*. Therefore, you are legally liable only for the written communication that you sign. Consequently, you should carefully and thoughtfully read and correct your written communication in a medical record *before* you ever sign it. If a nurse-author dictates or writes a hurried Nurses Note, which she or he signs without reading, it should not be surprising that glaring errors frequently appear in such a legal document and may cast doubt on the professionalism of the nurse-author. Nurse-writers need to make certain that there are no uncorrected spelling and/or typing errors in the legal records they author. Nurses need to be cognizant of the fact that uncorrected errors may create questions for readers about similar careless mistakes in a nurse's assessment and treatment of her or his patients. Killian (1991) states, "always make sure entries in the patient's record are legible and neat. Sloppy charting can lead to the inference that the nurse is a sloppy practitioner" (p. 22).

Conversely, however, when the nurse-author spends a few minutes considering the audience, purpose, and use for a particular record, edits the document for mistakes and misspelled words, and then carefully reviews the record's content and corrects any errors prior to signing it, the nurse-writer, the reader, and, ultimately, the patient all benefit.

Nurse-authors, like all writers of legal documents, need to understand that any misstatements, typos, and grammatical or spelling errors can be corrected and rewritten or retyped *prior to* signing the record, without any legal ramifications. If, however, the record needs to be altered *after* it has been signed by the nurse-author, then the nurse should *carefully* alter the legal document. First, any changes to a previously signed medical record should leave the original text visible beneath a single ink line that clearly demonstrates the incorrect wording or misstatement. All corrections should be legibly done in black ink and positioned above the incorrect word or words. Every correction must be initialed by the author and dated. In addition, it is a good practice to have a witness to the changes and the witness's initials and the date should also be included in the record.

It must be reiterated that correcting a *signed* medical record is not without potential legal risks and should be avoided if at all possible. The old adage, "an ounce of prevention is worth a pound of cure," is extremely applicable to this situation. If a nurse-author takes time to review a record and correct any inaccuracies before signing it, then there will be no need for post-signature corrections and possible legal complications at a later date.

Now that we've discussed the three stages of writing, let's look at one possible scenario you might encounter and use our knowledge about the prewriting, writing, and reviewing process to help us document the events and communication behaviors that occurred.

Example #17

Setting: A 20-year-old woman was admitted to the Labor Room at 1830 hours. Nurse Heidi Colb did an assessment, checked her fetal heart tones, evaluated her degree of dilatation, and reported her findings to Doctor Henry Jameson, the obstetrician who is on call for the patient's doctor, Martha Goode. By 2200 hours the patient is dilated 6 centimeters and is requesting an epidural anesthetic.

> *Ms. Lotus*: "I need an epidural, I can't take any more of this pain."
> *Nurse Colb*: "I've called Doctor Bijou, the anesthesiologist who's on call tonight, and he'll be here in just a couple of minutes."
> *Ms. Lotus*: "Oh my God, it hurts so bad!"

With that statement the patient suddenly rolled over, slammed against the plastic side-rail, which snapped into pieces, and the patient tumbled off the bed onto the floor. She did not lose consciousness. Nurse Colb pressed the emergency call button to summon help without leaving the patient's side. She questioned the patient about any areas of pain and assessed the patient quickly. Once help arrived, she got her back into bed. Following the incident, the patient's fetal heart tones, as well as the record on the fetal monitor, were unchanged. Nurse Colb notified Dr. Jameson of the patient's fall and her assessment.

The patient's labor progressed rapidly, and at 2300 hours the patient was taken to the Delivery Room and gave birth to a 9-pound 2-ounce boy. Both mother and baby were doing fine as Heidi Colb sat at the nurses' desk and began to consider how she was going to document the patient's fall, her assessment, interventions, communication of the event, and the patient's response to the accident.

In the space that follows, list the primary and secondary audiences that Nurse Colb should expect to use this particular medical record. Then list the different uses these diverse audiences have for such a record. Also, list the assessments and interventions that Nurse Colb needs to document to demonstrate that she was professionally competent and to persuade readers that she is both a credible nurse and nurse-author.

This particular incident would have as diverse a group of readers as any in nursing. Because of the nature of the incident, readers will need to know many details about the patient's condition prior to and following the incident, as well as the details of Nurse Colb's actions. (As you no doubt surmised, this incident has the potential to be catastrophic, either medically—for the patient and/or the baby—or legally—for the hospital, the doctor, and Nurse Colb.)

Most importantly, this medical record should meet the needs and expectations of Nurse Colb's peers and the patient's physician(s) who need to know exactly what happened, what the nurse's assessments of the patient's condition were before and after the incident, and how the nurse intervened to aid the patient following her fall. Similarly, the nursing supervisor, the hospital's risk management committee, Quality Assurance committee, and both nursing and hospital administrators would use this record to determine what happened, why it happened, how it could have been prevented, what steps were taken to prevent its occurrence, and what procedures need to be implemented to assure that a similar incident does not recur.

The hospital's and the physician's attorneys might use this record to assess the nurse-author's communication of the events that transpired as well as the nurse's account of her actions and communications with the patient, the patient's physician, and others. Finally, should the patient decide to sue, by inferring that the incident resulted from some malfeasance on the part of the nurse or the hospital, the patient's attorney would be interested in the information reported in this record.

With so many different users of this particular Nurses Note and so many diverse purposes for reading it, the nurse-author must not casually jot down a few cryptic sentences about the five hours she spent with the patient. This nurse-author needs to carefully evaluate, before he or she begins writing, what information is vital to, and expected by, these multifarious readers. The nurse-author of such a record would need to document what exactly happened, what precautions had been taken to prevent such an incident, his or her specific assessment of the patient following the incident, and the interventions undertaken to aid the patient after the fall. The nurse-author's communication with the patient, the patient's physician(s), other nursing staff, supervisors, and the patient's family, as well as the patient's post-fall condition must be scrupulously documented, including verbatim quotes whenever possible.

It is only after a nurse-author has analyzed his or her audience, evaluated their information needs and expectations for the particular Nurses Note he or she is authoring, and determined what facts, quotes, and impressions need to be reported, that the nurse-author is ready to begin writing his or her Nurses Notes about the incident, event, or outcome.

Two examples of Nurses Notes that attempt to document the above scenario, beginning at 2200 hours, follow. (Remember, there are many ways to present the information that is needed and expected by an audience, your role as a professional nurse is to find the method that best informs readers and persuades them about your competency and credibility.)

Example A

2200 hrs.:   Patient had a contriction (sic) and rolled around on the bed until she fell to the floor. She didn't lose consciousness and she didn't complain of any pain, except in her gluteal area.

2230 hrs.:   Dr. Jameson and Dr. Bijou in to see patient. Epidural anesthetic given. Patient's vital signs and fetal heart tone are ok.

2255 hrs.:   Fully dilated moved to Delivery.

2311 hrs.:   Vaginal delivery of 9.2 pound boy with APGER (sic) of 9.

2335 hrs.:   Mother and baby returned to Room 512.

HEIDI COLB, R.N.

This is a flawed, "bare-bones" record. A reader is provided enough information to tell that the patient and baby survived some type of incident, but there are no specifics about the event, the patient's response to the event, or the baby's response to it. In addition, there are spelling errors (contriction, APGER) that further cheapen the value of this document for the reader and demonstrate that either Nurse Colb didn't take the time to reread this brief record before she signed it, or she wasn't competent enough to know how to spell common medical terms. In either case, this document calls into question the nurse's professional competency and credibility and when a nurse is involved in a potentially libelous incident he or she does not need to cast doubt on his or her expertise.

Compare the record in Example A with the record that follows:

Example B

2200 hrs.:   Ms. Lotus was having contractions about two minutes apart. The fetal heart rate was 148. The patient had an apparent contraction, and, while screaming in pain she rolled abruptly onto her left side and struck the side rail that was raised to prevent her from rolling off the bed. However, the left side rail broke off and the patient rolled about two feet from the bed to the floor. She landed on her gluteal area and did not strike her head or her abdomen. I was standing a few feet from the patient dialing Dr. Jameson to tell him that Dr. Bijou was coming up to start the epidural when the patient screamed and tumbled to the floor. She had no loss of consciousness. I asked Ms. Lotus if she hurt anywhere and she replied, "my butt is a little sore, but that's all."

2205 hrs.:   After pressing the emergency buzzer, I made the patient rest on the floor until nurses Mary Beth O'Connor and Billie May Britton arrived to help get the patient into a new bed with intact side rails. While the other nurses checked the patient's vital signs, I used the doppler and checked the fetal heart rate that was 149. Ms. Lotus's pulse before the fall had been 92 and it was still 92 afterwards, her blood pressure was unchanged at 124/80, and her respirations had increased slightly from 20 before the fall to 24 after-wards. She had clear breath sounds throughout both lungs. I then notified Dr. Jameson about the incident and Ms. Lotus's vital signs, fetal heart rate, and that she was alert and well oriented and not complaining of any pain, except her labor which continued with hard contractions 2 minutes apart. Dr. Jameson did not give any new orders. I then notified Celia Horn, the Labor Room Charge Nurse, and Beth Mendenhall, the evening supervisor, about the patient's fall and her condition.

2220 hrs.:   The patient's breath sounds remain clear, her heart rate is regular and unchanged. Her abdomen is soft, except during her [contractions], and she had normal active bowel sounds and no abdominal tenderness except with her contractions.

2230 hrs.:   Dr. Jameson arrived and examined the patient who denies any complaints except her labor. Dr. Bijou administered the epidural.

2245 hrs.:   Ms. Lotus states, "I'm much better, that was good stuff he put in there."

2255 hrs.:   Dr. Jameson notified that the patient is completely dilated and fully effaced. Patient transferred to the Delivery Room.

2311 hrs.:   Patient had a vaginal delivery of a 9 lb., 2 oz. boy
               without difficulty. [APGAR was 9.]
2335 hrs.:   Ms. Lotus and her baby out of the Delivery Room
               without any problems and returned to Room 512 for
               rooming-in. The infant's APGAR was 10 when
               taken from the Delivery Room.

HEIDI COLB, R.N.

While Example A does provide some information, it could hardly
be relied upon if the nurse-author, the physician, or the hospital
needed it to demonstrate what occurred and what actions were
taken, and how the patient and the fetus/infant responded. There
may be rare instances where a patient's labor and delivery are so
routine and uneventful that a smattering of information is all that
is needed to meet the expectations of medical and extra-medical
readers. However, an event as potentially catastrophic as the one
described in the above scenario must be evaluated and communicated with a much greater attention to detail and an awareness of
the possible legal as well as medical uses for such a record. Most
important, how could Nurse Colb's peers have used Example A to
help them determine anything about the patient's or the fetus's
response to the incident? If the patient hadn't delivered before the
end of Nurse Colb's shift, could her replacement have used Example
A to evaluate any changes in the patient's condition? Could nursing
supervisors or administrators have used this example to support
their belief that proper precautions had been taken? Could Nurse
Colb, three or four years later, have relied on Example A to aid her
memory of the event and to demonstrate that she was a competent,
compassionate, and credible professional nurse? If your answer to
any or all of these questions is no, then you are well on your way to
understanding the importance of careful, clear, and complete documentation. The portion of Example B that is surrounded by brack-
ets illustrates the information Nurse Colb added *after* she read her
note, and *before* she signed the document. As we stated earlier, it is
completely legal and extremely important for you to review your
written communication and make any necessary corrections, as
Nurse Colb did to the misspelled word "contrictions," *before* you
sign the record.

Example B demonstrates how the nurse-author used the writing process to provide a detailed account of the incident for a variety of medical and extra-medical readers (administrators, insurance companies, medical records reviewers, and lawyers), and at the same time demonstrated her professional competency in dealing with the unexpected event and her credibility in assessing, intervening, and reporting the incident. As a reader of Example B, you should be able to determine that the nurse-author took great pains to ensure that a reader's questions and concerns about the incident and the staffs' responses to it were addressed and answered. For example, this record not only reports that the rails were up, but also that a new bed was used after the fall to prevent a recurrence. In addition, the nurse- author uses language choices that did not aggravate the nature of the event. The author uses "tumbled" instead of fell. Tumbled connotes a much more gentle act—people fall from a roof, but they generally tumble off a bed. The nurse tells readers that she used the emergency buzzer to summon help, thereby inferring that she never left the patient's side. She documented who assisted her, what information was communicated from her to the patient, the physician, and the supervisory staff. In so doing, the nurse-author clearly demonstrates her understanding of her role as both a health care provider and a communicator and at the same time persuades readers that she is a highly competent and extremely credible nursing professional.

It may take a few (very few) extra minutes to prewrite, write, and review the Nurses Notes you author, but the enormous benefits you reap in terms of demonstrating your competency and credibility, and the vital role you play in assisting your peers, other health care team members, and the patient's physician(s) in assessing and evaluating the patient's condition and response to treatment, should make any brief inconvenience seem trivial indeed.

Chapter 6 is intended to further assist you in learning how to utilize the writing process so that you can clearly and effectively communicate written information that both apprises readers of the patient's condition and persuades them to view the nurse-author as a competent and credible professional nurse.

6

Written Communication
in Nursing

RATIONALE

As we discussed in Chapter 5, you write in order to communicate with someone other than yourself. Except for private diaries, the only reason to write something is to share it with someone else. In health care, written communication is shared among dozens, sometimes hundreds, of people, many of whom the author never knows. As vast as this potential audience is, however, an author of a medical record must still anticipate the reader's needs and expectations and attempt to ensure that her or his written document meets or exceeds the various readers' needs. For years countless writers have described the perils and importance of charting in a medical record (Afflerbach, 1986; Connaway, 1985; Cuzzell, 1986; Dobberstein, 1986; Feutz, 1987; Gondringer, 1986; Harkins, 1986; Iyer, 1991a, 1991b; Jacob, 1985; Manion, 1986; Philpott, 1986; Rhodes, 1986; Rutkowski, 1985; Thornton, 1986; Weeks & Darrah, 1985).

DOCUMENTATION

As most nursing textbooks and nursing journals proclaim, patient care is not complete until you have carefully and precisely communicated in writing about the patient's condition and care. While it is true that numerous authors have discussed the perils of documentation and the importance of defensive record-keeping (see the list of authors above), few, if any, of these writers have provided a process that can be used to author medical records. Most of the recommendations concern strategies, formats, and content, but almost no one discusses the methods you can use to evaluate the audience's needs and expectations, your writing, and the way to revise that writing to meet both the reader's needs and your own.

Prewriting

As we discussed in Chapter 5, prewriting allows you to assess your reader's needs and expectations and to determine what information you should provide in order to meet those requirements. (Remember—it is a nurse-author's responsibility to meet the needs of a reader, not vice versa.)

In some ways you are lucky that you need to communicate primarily in only one format—Nurses Notes—though the intricacies and demands of this record should probably discourage any jubilation.

Let's take a minute to quickly review the *primary audience* for Nurses Notes. These readers include, but are not limited to:

1. *Your peers,* who use your record to evaluate: the patient's condition while you were caring for her or him; the treatment the patient received; the results, if any, from any interventions; any changes in the patient's condition during the time you cared for her or him; any unusual or unanticipated events that had an impact on the patient's condition, future condition, or treatment; your assessment of the patient's condition (including both your subjective and objective findings); and any changes to your nursing diagnoses.

2. *The patient's physician, consultants, and other members of the health care team,* all of whom want to know the same basic information that your peers require from the document.

These two primary audiences have diverse levels of medical education (from a respiratory or physical therapist, to a dietitian, to nurses, and physicians), yet they all can be expected to know basic medical terminology and some medical jargon, while many of the secondary readers for these records cannot be expected to possess similar education and technical knowledge.

The *secondary audience* for Nurses Notes include, but are not limited to:

1. *Nursing supervisors,* who use these records to evaluate your patient care, communication skills, adherence to policy and procedures, quality assurance, and documentation. These supervisors also frequently use the medical record in determining the level of promotion or salary increase a professional nurse should receive.

2. *Hospital administrators and risk managers* occasionally review your written communication to evaluate a patient's or physician's complaint and to determine if any legal liability has occurred (as in Example #14 in Chapter 4 in which a patient fell and suffered a subdural hematoma).

3. *Infection control officers and Quality Assurance personnel* review Nurses Notes to obtain information about postoperative and nosocomical infections and for utilization in Q.A. committees and studies.

4. *Hospital financial clerks* frequently review these records to determine if patients have been charged for all of the services and products that were provided.

5. *Medical records personnel* use the Nurses Notes to aid in DRG assessment, discharge planning, and Peer Review.

6. *JCAHO and Peer Review Organizations (PRO)* use Nurses Notes to evaluate the hospital's adherence to regulations, as well as the patient's condition at the time of admission, the treatment the patient received, the patient's response to that treatment, and the patient's condition at the time of discharge. While it is true that these reviewers use the physician's records as the primary documentation of a patient's hospitalization, it is often the Nurses Notes that supply the corroborating or clarifying information frequently needed by reviewers.

7. *Nursing students* often use these records to learn about a patient's illness, treatment, nursing assessment, and diagnosis. In

addition, the students can use these documents as models for their own written communication.

8. *Malpractice attorneys* use Nurses Notes to evaluate the care and treatment a patient received as well as a means to compare a nurse's assessment and statements about a patient with a physician's written communication about the same incident or patient.

Armed with this knowledge about the audience, purpose, and use for these documents, you can now begin to decide what information is beneficial and important to readers and what information is trite and routine. For example, it is not necessary to document if the side-rails are up or down on every hospitalized patient; however, on children, elderly, cognitively impaired, or heavily medicated patients, it would make good sense to demonstrate your competency in preventive nursing by a simple statement that the bed rails were up.

Similarly, it would not be necessary to record in the Nurses Notes that a patient ate all of his or her meal (since this information is usually recorded on the graphics sheet), unless the patient has not been eating or was not supposed to be eating and did it anyway. The point is that Nurses Notes will become redundant and useless for readers if they merely re-record nonessential information that can be found elsewhere in the chart. Yet, sometimes, it is very important to re-record information in order to assure that readers are aware of it and to demonstrate your credibility and competency in providing it for them.

Let's look at some examples of Nurses Notes. We will use your rewrite of the scenario that opened this book, Example #1, as the basis for a Nurses Note about the interaction. We will assume that the patient had an uneventful 1500-2300 (3-11) hours, therefore use the space below for your Nurses Note.

As you thought about writing your record of Mr. Swenson's care, what questions did you ask yourself? Did you consider the value of Mr. Swenson's anxiety for readers? Were you concerned about the need to communicate your responses (as the nurse) to Mr. Swenson's anxious behaviors? Or did you feel that Nurse O'Hara was correct in not documenting their interaction?

If you concurred with Nurse O'Hara's noncommunication about the event, go to page one of this text and begin reading again. If you disagreed with her noncommunication, then we are on our way to helping you become a more effective communicator of written information. We hope you recognized the importance, for your peers, the anesthetist or anesthesiologist, and the surgeon, of Mr. Swenson's anxiety. While it is true that most patients experience preoperative anxiety, Mr. Swenson's was more intense than most. Without reassurance from his nurse, this anxiety might have caused him severe stress or even the cancellation of his operation.

Any event that you, as a professional nurse, deem to be unusual, potentially dangerous (medically or psychosocially), or a legal liability should be carefully and completely documented in the patient's medical record. The reason for Supervisor Yancey's anger in Example #14 is the lack of documentation in the patient's chart of the potentially libelous fall that resulted in a life-threatening injury to the patient. The fact that the incident and its results are not recorded until hours after the event and the resulting treatment makes the documentation legally suspect and less credible than it would have been if it were recorded immediately after the event and then followed by detailed evaluations of the patient's condition, changes in his or her assessment, eventual tests, surgery, and response to the treatment.

Let's examine the following eight hours of documentation about an actual patient in a JCAHO hospital. This record was authored, in pen, by an R.N. This document and all of the Nurses Notes in this chapter, are recorded verbatim from the medical record, the only exception being that the records for clarity and publication are typed.

Record #4

4/16/91

0800: Awake, eating breakfast. Oriented x 3, skin W/D, no S.O.B. noted O2 off. Crackles noted RML and crackles noted on LLL. Abd. soft with active BS. HLN intact to LFA site clear. Pedal pulses + bilat. Resp-nonlabored. No complaints.

1000: Family here to visit patient

1100: Up (up arrow in original record) to BR, gait steady.

1200: Ate well. Bath done.

1300: Ate lunch well.

1400: SR UP (up arrow in original record) & call light in reach wanting to take a nap.

[Abbreviations apparently represent: W/D = warm and dry; S.O.B.= shortness of breath; RML = right middle lobe; LLL = left lower lobe; Abd. = abdomen; BS (can be breath sounds, but here = bowel sounds; HLN = heparin lock needle; LFA = left forearm; BR (can be bedrails), but here appears to be bathroom; SR = side rails]

Please answer the following questions about Record #4.

1. What care, treatments, etc., did this nurse provide to the patient during the eight hours that are supposed to be reported in this document?

_____

_____

2. How is the patient responding to treatment and what treatment is the patient receiving?

_____

_____

3. Are the crackles in the patient's lungs new or different from her breath sounds 24 hours earlier or a week ago when she was admitted?

_____

4. Do the numerous abbreviations aid your understanding of this document or distract you?

_____

5. Did the patient have pedal edema?

_____

6. Why do you think the nurse-author of Record #4 documented the patient's pedal pulses?

_____

_____

7. The assessment of the patient's eating is recorded at 1200 and again at 1300, why?

_____

8. The patient's O2 is reported to be off. Is it ordered to be: off, prn, or on?

_____

Isn't it frightening how a simple half-page Nurses Note can cause a reader so much confusion, call into question the competency and professional credibility of the nurse-author, and provide almost no useful information about the patient's condition, treatment, or response to that treatment?

Let's carefully dissect and analyze Record #4 in order to aid our understanding, from both a writer and reader's perspective, of the communication that occurs or does not occur in the document. Remember, the only reason to write is to communicate, and, as a writer, you must assume that the reader is not going to call you up or track you down in order to get an explanation for your writing. One big advantage speakers have over writers is the use of nonverbal behaviors. Speakers can use listeners' nonverbal behaviors as cues to the audience's understanding and acceptance of her or his other message. Writers, however, do not have such a luxury. You can only rely on your own assessment of the record and your comparison between what you believe the audience for the document needs and expects and what you think the document communicates.

Record #4 provides a reader with no specific information about the patient who is described. It is true that the document bears an imprint at the top of the page that is supposed to identify this patient by name and hospital number; however, we have all heard and seen examples of patients whose charts had other people's records incorrectly assembled with someone else's; and it is not uncommon for a clerk to stamp the wrong patient's name on a medical record, include it in the chart, and everyone fill it out without ever checking to see whose name appears on the top of the form. Therefore, once a shift identify your patient by name in the Nurses Notes. It makes you appear more empathic and caring—you know the patient's name and use it—plus it assures that in a worst-case scenario, should the chart get confused, doused with Betadine or coffee, or even partially burned in a fire, your record will help to identify this document as belonging to a particular person, and not just one more collection of remarks and abbreviations about an unnamed individual.

With that in mind, is the patient discussed in Record #4 a male or female? You can't tell from this record. While it may not seem to be important, the fact is that you are reporting your interactions with another human being for eight hours of her or his life and, yet, not once is that person identified in any way other than an anatomical, dietary, or physiological state. It would be hard to make a case in court that a nurse was very compassionate, concerned, or caring if she or he doesn't even have the courtesy, not to mention the wisdom, to identify the patient who is being described for numerous readers.

Let's look at the record, line by line. If the patient is eating breakfast, does it not automatically follow that she or he is awake. If so, then why mention it? Since the time is recorded as 0800 for all of the statements until 1000 hours, are we to assume that the patient was awake and eating breakfast while the nurse was doing her assessment, listening to the patient's lungs, checking his or her abdomen and IV, and evaluating her or his pedal pulses. It's no wonder the patient didn't complain; she was eating and according to this record she ate well until 1200, took a short break, and then ate well again until 1300.

We realize that sarcasm has almost no place in the evaluation of written communication, yet it should aid us in pointing out how carelessly this record was created. We said earlier in this chapter that your peers, physicians, and other health care team members use this document. Do you believe that this record offers much information that could assist those readers in caring for this patient? If your answer is no, then the nurse-author of this Nurses Note failed in his or her attempt at communicating effectively with readers.

Let's rethink or revise Record #4 and see if we can't find better language choices and a more persuasive method to document the eight hours of care that was provided for this patient.

Record #5

4/16/91

0800: Mr. Tupperman is sitting up in bed, waiting for breakfast, Lasix and Lanoxin given. He commented, "I feel so much better today, I'm starving." He is breathing without difficulty and his prn oxygen was not in use. His vital signs were within normal limits and his skin is warm and dry; he is oriented times three and his breath sounds contain crackles in both the RML and LLL, but they are less intense than 24 hours ago, and there are no wheezes, which were present last p.m. His heart sounds and bowel sounds are normal, he has 1+ pedal edema bilaterally, which is less than yesterday, and pedal pulses are 2+ and equal bilaterally. His heparin lock needle is intact in the LFA without redness or swelling.

0900:   His family is visiting and he ambulated to the bathroom by himself without difficulty.

1030:   Mr. Tupperman went by wheelchair to get his chest X-ray and EKG.

1230:   He is sitting up at the bedside eating and has no complaints of pain or shortness of breath.

1400:   Mr. Tupperman voided 422 ccs of straw-colored urine this eight hours and had 710 ccs of oral intake. He is sleeping with the side rails up and his call light within easy reach.

If you compare Record #5 with Record #4 you should see some obvious differences. Record #5 is not a collection of cryptic notations and abbreviations; instead, it carefully describes eight hours of hospitalization for a particular patient, Mr. Tupperman. Record #5 identifies the specific patient who is being discussed, the patient's subjective assessment of his condition in his own words, the nurse's objective and subjective assessment (no wheezes today, less intense crackles, and decreased pedal edema), the tests and treatments he received, and the results of the treatment (pulse is within normal range and his urine output is adequate for someone on a diuretic). Record #5 avoids the redundancy of quantifying his eating and it does not report that the patient is awake because readers know that he is awake since he is eating and talking. Finally, the nurse-author of Record #5 carefully documents his or her nursing assessment, treatments, and interventions so that a reader can be assured that the nurse is competent and credible, both as a nurse and as a communicator. After reading both of these examples, ask yourself which record provides you with clear, descriptive information about the patient's condition, intervention, response to treatment, and nursing assessment, and which does not? The answer should encourage you to continue reading and to work on communicating in a medical record like the author of Record #5 instead of the author of Record #4.

The following record is a verbatim transcription of an anonymous medical record.

Record #6

Home Health Skilled Nurse Visit
Report/Progress Notes

1. **Date**:_5-23-91_____
2. **Patient**:_____
3. **Acct.#**:_____
4. **Address**:_____
5. **Doctor**:_____
6. **Diagnosis**:_Urinary retention_____
7. **Vital Signs**: Temp_97.2_ Pulse_82_ Resp._18_ B/P_116/72_
8. **Chest Auscultations**: _X_Clear
9. **Dyspnea**: _X_ None
10. **Cough**: _X_None ___Moist ___Dry ___ Productive
    ___Nonproductive
11. **Edema**: _X_None
12. **Medications**: _X_None _ as Rx's—administered by son____
13. **Dressings**: X None
14. **Drainage**:_X_None Amount: _small _medium _large
15. **Genitourinary**: ___ No problems _____
16. **Catheter**: _ None _ patent _ nonpatent upon time of visit
    _X_inserted _ replaced Catheter No._____
    Bulb size ___ Irrigated ___
17. **GI**: _X_No problems
18. **Diet**:_Reg. as tol._ Eating _X_ Well ___ Fair ___ Poor
19. **Patient Attitude**: ___receptive ___non-receptive
    _X_cooperative ___ uncooperative

Continued

Record #6 (Continued)

20. ___ Oriented   X Confused

21. **Teaching and training:** _____

_____

22. **Activity Status:** ambulates unassisted-gait steady, does
      hold to walls to steady self _____

23. **Home Health Aide Supervisory Visit:** ___ yes ___no

24. **Phone call to physician:** _____

25. **Orders received:** _____

_____

26. **Remarks:** SNV [Skilled nurse visit] to cath for residual. After
      vdg unmeasured amt in BR cathed with #14 straight without
      diff using sterile tech. 250 cc clear yellow urine returned. Tol
      procedure well. Denies any problems or discomfort.

SIGNATURE:_____

If you examine Record #6 closely you will see that readers
have very little specific information about this patient and this
home health visit. We are not told if this is the first home health
visit or if the patient is routinely seen for another problem. In
fact, readers cannot determine from this record who diagnosed
the patient's urinary retention. For example, many patients
complain about an inability to void or a feeling that they can't
completely empty their bladders, but this record does not communicate any information about the specifics of the "urinary
retention." In addition, readers might be perplexed to learn that
the patient, who is described by a check mark on this form as
confused, "voided an unmeasured amt in BR." As medically
trained readers, you know that the only way to catheterize a
patient "for residual" is to determine if, and how much urine
the patient voided prior to catheterization. In this case the
nurse-author did not obtain, for whatever reason, a voided
specimen and, consequently, a reader must question the valid-
ity of the procedure as well as the competency of the nurse who
performs and reports it. If the patient is confused, how do we
know he or she even voided, or, for that matter, how did the
nurse know? Again this overly simplistic document fails to

communicate the information readers need to assess what was done for the patient, why it was done, and what the purpose of the test was. There is no mention of treatment for the patient's "retained" 250cc of urine. So, readers must wonder why she or he was catheterized. There is no record that the physician was notified, or that she or he will be notified. In short, this document is ineffective in communicating even the most basic information that readers need and expect about this patient's condition and treatment. Furthermore, the brevity and lack of information in this document call into question, not only the nurse's competency and professional credibility, but also the Home Health agency that created this form and allows such records to be maintained.

In all likelihood this patient has a chart at the Home Health office that provides additional information about this patient's cognitive status, the reason for this visit, and perhaps even the interventions that are planned, but the problem is that each medical record you author is a *singular* document that is supposed to stand alone. You should not create a record and assume that a reader will have other records available to explain, define, or reinforce your writing. The only purpose for creating a medical record is to communicate information and if the *singular* document does not accomplish that, then it is ineffective and may demonstrate malfeasance or at the very least professional incompetency on your part.

We can use Record #6 to aid us in learning about effective written communication. In the space that follows, rewrite Record #6 and attempt to communicate what the patient's problem was that necessitated this treatment, your nursing diagnoses, your actions, the results of those actions, and your planned interventions. Feel free to create whatever information you need to make this an effective form of written communication.

We have discussed the numerous problems with flow sheet formats and both the 8-hour shift of a 24-hour flow sheet in Chapter 5 and Record #6 demonstrate the difficulties that flow sheets cause for writers and readers. As a writer, you feel successful if you check the appropriate boxes and make some mundane comment about any abnormal reports. As a reader, however, you can see that the time it takes to scan a flow sheet and derive the necessary information is compounded by the lack of explanation, description, and evaluation. A reader of Record #6 cannot determine what the patient complained of, the specific reason for the catheterization for residual urine, or the treatment plan based on the findings from the catheterization. Therefore, the major reasons for authoring the record have not been fulfilled and, consequently, the reader must ask what is the value of this document to the present and future care of this patient? (We hope your rewrites took these negative aspects into account and improved on the record.)

One possible rewrite of Record #6 follows:

Record #7

5/23/91

I was called by Mr. Jenson's son and informed, "dad seems to be going to the bathroom every few minutes." Dr. Munie was notified and ordered catheterization for residual and a UA. The patient was alert and oriented when I went to the house and he was cooperative with my assessment and catheterization and followed my instructions without difficulty. His pulse was 82, respirations were 18, blood pressure was 116/72 and his temperature was 97.2. His lungs were clear and his abdomen was soft with no suprapubic tenderness, but there was some fullness. Mr. Jenson's son helped him void about 35 ccs of light yellow urine. I placed a 14 french catheter without difficulty and 250 ccs of straw-colored urine was evacuated/drained. He tolerated the procedure without significant discomfort. Dr. Munie was notified of the residual and requested that the catheter be left in to gravity, he called Bactrim-DS bid for ten days into the pharmacy and a urinalysis and culture were done on the cath specimen and I took them to the Med Arts Lab. I will recheck Mr. Jenson in 48 hours and I have advised his son to call me or Dr. Munie if Mr. Jenson develops any high fever, nausea and vomiting, or becomes severely ill.

Nursing Diagnoses:	**Interventions:**
1. Alteration in urinary elimination	a. catheterized with 14 fr., to gravity drainage.
	b. keep daily record of intake & output.
2. Potential for infection	a. instructed son on care of catheter & cleansing.
	b. review catheter care procedure with son in 48 hrs.
	c. take temperature BID & record.
	d. son taught signs and symptoms of urinary tract infection & instructed to notify Dr. if outside parameters.

This record attempts to communicate descriptive information about the patient's condition, the plans for assessing the patient's complaints, the patient's response to the catheterization, and the treatment plans and follow-up evaluations. Record #7 is a narrative, not a flow sheet. Yet, you should have no trouble in discerning all of the information that was provided in Record #6, but in a format and style that is easier to read and evaluate.

Record #7 also provides information about the patient and his complaint. Readers know why the nurse was asked to "cath for residual." In addition, this nurse-author chooses to use the first person, "I," when describing her actions. Contrary to traditional record-keeping practices of using a third-person removed narrator, the use of the first person allows a reader to see the nurse-author's personal involvement in the patient's assessment and care. In addition, there is no question about who catheterized the patient, ordered the treatment, and carried out the interventions. If you have trouble following this logic, reread Records #4, 5, 6, and 7. After you finish each document, make a note of your responses to the use of third-person removed versus first person communication. Ask yourself, when Record #4 states, "no SOB noted," who did the evaluation? Was it the patient who did not note any shortness of breath, or was it a family member, nurse aide, or the nurse-author?

Do not be afraid to use personal pronouns to describe your actions and try, whenever possible, to quote verbatim the patient's or the patient's family's statements when these reports can enhance a reader's understanding and assessment of your actions and the patient's treatment. Let's see if the next record can help us explain why the patient's own words are often very helpful in communicating information for readers of the medical record.

Record #8

Emergency Room Record

NURSING REPORT

Allergies: ASA
Temp.: _____   **Resp.:** _28_
Pulse: _100_   **B/P:** _140/90_
Condition on admission: __ Good _X_ Fair __ Poor __ Other
Brief History: Diving into shallow water and cut top of head. Cold. Knows that he is in the hospital & that friend brought him here. Doesn't know what town he is in.

Current Medications: none

Please answer the following questions about this verbatim transcription of an actual E.R. record.

1. Was the patient unconscious after the injury?

   yes _____   unsure _____   no _____

2. This patient arrived at the E.R. at 0500 hours. When did the accident occur?

   _____

3. Had the patient been drinking or using drugs? _____

4. What were the dimensions of the "cut"? _____cm.

5. Anatomically, where is the "top of head" located?

   ___ hairline at the forehead
   ___ temple
   ___ occiput
   ___ base of skull
   ___ other

6. Did the patient have any numbness, paralysis, or neck pain from diving into shallow water and hitting his head?

   yes _____   unsure _____   no _____

One of the most critical forms of Nurses Notes is the Emergency Room Record. This document is frequently used as the basis for determining malfeasance and malpractice in post-trauma and urgent-care situations. Record #8 presents numerous problems for medical readers and potentially serves as a legal liability for the nurse-author and the physician who treated this patient.

Let's suppose that five minutes after arriving in the E.R. this patient develops some numbness in his arms and legs, and, by the time he's sutured, he is unable to move his extremities. How could the nurse-author of this record use it to demonstrate that he or she did a thorough interview and assessment of the patient? He or she could not use the record to demonstrate it, and by the time the case went to trial, two, three, or four years after the patient presented to the E.R., the nurse's memory would probably not aid her or him either.

Or, what if the patient arrived in the E.R. and after a few minutes developed some confusion and became increasingly lethargic, went into a coma, and died. Could the nurse use this document to demonstrate his or her assessment and the information he or she communicated to the E.R. physician about the patient?

You should be able to deduce the dangers of this type of careless record-keeping and poor communication. In the space below, rewrite Record #8, but try to supply enough information so that a reader can determine what you learned about the patient's condition, what you did for the patient, and how she or he responded.

Emergency Room Record

NURSING REPORT

Allergies: ASA
Temp.: _____   **Resp.:** _28_
Pulse: _100_   **B/P:** _140/90_
Condition on admission: __Good   _X_ Fair __Poor __Other
Brief History: _____

_____

_____

_____

Current medications: none

Some of the key elements that needed to be in your rewrite include the patient's own statement about exactly what happened. If he or she can't provide that information, try to obtain it from someone who was with the patient and then identify, in the record, the source of the information. Whenever possible, use direct quotes from the source of the information, and, especially, use the patient's own words to quantify the amount of drugs or alcohol that has been consumed. If you disagree with the patient's statement, follow the patient's quote with a simple statement such as, "In spite of the patient's insistence that he hasn't been drinking his breath smells of alcohol, he is slurring his speech, and his friend states, 'we've had about 12 beers apiece.' " This additional subjective and objective data may come in handy if there are questions at a later date about the patient's mental state in the E.R. In addition, such quotes from patients, families, and friends prevent your having to make subjective judgments about the patient's level of intoxication or impairment, which is difficult to support without blood and/or urine tests. However, your statement that the patient smells of alcohol combined with a quote from a friend should demonstrate to any supervisor, physician, lawyer, or jury that this patient is not being honest with you and is more than likely under the influence of drugs or alcohol.

Now, let's rewrite this record (we have the E.R. physician's documentation of this patient's visit to the E.R. to help us), so we can see just how different that information is from the nurse-author's descriptions in Record #8.

Record #9

Emergency Room Record

NURSING REPORT

Allergies: ASA
Temp.: ___ **Resp.**: 28
Pulse: 100 **B/P**: 140/90

Continued

Record #9 (Continued)

Condition on admission: __Good   _X_ Fair __Poor __Other

Brief History: This 17-year-old white male was diving into the lake from the shore. At approximately 0400 hrs he jumped in and hit his head on some rocks. He denies any loss of consciousness or any numbness in his extremities. He denies any neck pain. He is alert and oriented to time, place, and person. He is bleeding from a gaping 20 cm. laceration that extends across his scalp from the left temple region to the right. He denies any other complaints. His last tetanus shot was in 1985. Dr. Hitch was notified and the wound was cleansed with Betadine. The patient states, "I've only had three beers all night." His mother brought the patient to the E.R. and signed his consent for treatment.

Current medications: none

The E.R. physician reported in her or his record that the laceration, described by the nurse-author in Record #8 as "cut top of head," to in fact be a laceration that extended across the entire scalp from ear to ear. The patient had been drinking, had no numbness or neck pain, and had not lost consciousness. As you compare Record #9 with #8 you should be amazed by the enormity of differences between the two, and yet this is the same patient that is being described. Written communication can be a great asset or it can be a terrible liability. Think about how the discrepancies between the nurse's statements in Record #8 and those in Record #9 would confuse and frustrate a reader. Such confusion is unlikely to occur, however, when you are thorough and carefully document the who, what, where, why, when, and how of each patient's visit. You should describe who the patient is, why he or she is at the hospital, what happened to her or him, when it happened, where she or he hurts, and how she or he compares this pain with other pain they've experienced (less than root canal, greater than child birth, etc.).

Let's use this kind of description and return to Example #12 from Chapter 4.

Example #12

Nurse Jackson: "Hello, Dr. Bowers, this is Canera Jackson, I'm on three-West at County General and I'm concerned about your patient Mr. Lumbata in Room 373. He's called me down to his room twice in the past half-hour to complain about his abdomen hurting. He says it's the worst pain he's ever felt."

Dr. Bowers: "Isn't he the patient that was admitted with chest pain and anxiety?"

Nurse Jackson: "yes, but . . ."

Dr. Bowers: "Well, I wouldn't get too worked up about his complaints—he's probably just anxious again. Give him five milligrams of Valium p.o. and see if that doesn't fix his bellyache."

Nurse Jackson: "O.K., but . . ."

We are going to assume that the nurse carried out the doctor's order and gave the patient Valium 5 mg p.o. In the space that follows write a Nurses Note about the patient's pain, your notification of the physician, the treatment ordered, the patient's response to that treatment, your nursing diagnoses, assessments, and interventions. You may assume the Valium did not ease the patient's pain and that the nurse called the physician back after about 30 minutes.

As you no doubt surmised and we discussed in Chapter 4, the conversation in Example #12 posed a difficult transactional communication problem for Nurse Jackson, but it posed an even greater written communication dilemma for the nurse. Here is a true legal nightmare. The nurse must document what the patient told her about his complaint, what she assessed as the patient's problem, what she communicated to the doctor, and what the doctor ordered. However, she needs to do all of this without accusing anyone of malpractice or malfeasance, but she must be sure to document everything to ensure that a reader knows what the nurse's assessment was, what she did, why she did it, the results of her actions, and her follow-up actions.

Record #10

Nurses Notes

1/27/91

1500:   Mr. Lumbata has a three hour history of substernal and epigastric pain. He is resting comfortably and vital signs are within normal limits. Telemetry shows normal sinus rhythm, only complaint is of some slight epigastric pain. Denies any chest pain or shortness of breath.

1745:   The patient refuses his supper because, "I feel sick to my stomach." He also refuses Dramamine. Vital signs and temperature at 1730 hours within normal limits.

1900:   Called to patient's room, "I'm having the worst pain in my stomach I've ever had in my life." He is diaphoretic, pulse—124, respirations—22, BP—106/66 and his temperature is 101.3. I notified Dr. Bowers of the patient's complaints, diaphoresis, and vital signs. He ordered Valium 5 mg. p.o.

1910:   Valium 5 mg. p.o. given.

1935:   Patient continues to complain of pain, "That pill didn't help!" Pulse—135, BP—98/58.

1940:   I called Dr. Bowers and informed him of the patient's changing vital signs and nonrelief of pain from the

Valium. He ordered a CBC, lytes, BUN, Creatinine, CPK, CKMB, EKG, and flat and upright abdominal X-ray.

1945: Lab tests obtained, IV of Lactated Ringers increased to 150 cc/hr.

1955: Patient distended and without bowel sounds for one minute, BP—90/50. Dr. Bowers at bedside.

2005: Patient prepped for emergency laparotomy.

2010: BP—60/0, P—150, R—32. Type-specific blood ordered.

2012: Patient arrested, CPR initiated. Dr. Bowers, myself, Marty Jonsen, R.N., Helen Tootie, R.N., and Brad Metner, R.T.—code team. A second IV was started with Dopamine 800 mg. in 500 ccs of D5W. Epinephrine 1 mg. IV was given twice, he was defibrillated three times starting with 200 joules and increasing to 250 and then 300 without success.

2029: Dr. Bowers pronounced the patient dead and informed the family. The family refused an autopsy.

2049: The body was released at the family's request to Golden Pines Funeral Home.

Record #10 documents an unexpected death and communicates the events that transpired from 1500 hours when Nurse Jackson first saw Mr. Lumbata until the patient expired and his body was sent to the funeral home. This record does not attempt to evaluate the nurse or physician's actions, orders, or treatment. That is not the purpose for creating Nurses Notes. Instead, the record details the patient's condition, the changes that occurred in the patient's condition, the nurse's response to those changes, the doctor's response to the nurse's phone calls, the tests and treatments that were ordered, and the patient's eventual demise. It is vitally important that nurses always document their actions and communications meticulously. Such documentation serves as testimony to the nurse's actions and professional competence, and eventually may be used to demonstrate her or his credibility. Conversely, a poor record-keeper might be accused of being a poor nurse and/or a poor transactional communicator. (Either or which could be detrimental to a patient or in a court of law.)

What Nurse Jackson does not want is for the doctor or a lawyer to intimate that she might not have effectively communicated the patient's illness to Dr. Bowers. A carelessly written record might be used as support for such a claim, but an effectively authored Nurses Note that demonstrates what the nurse knew, what she communicated, and how she responded is invaluable days, weeks, months, or even years later when someone might be trying to determine exactly what was communicated to Dr. Bowers.

Written communication is vital to the exchange of information between health care professionals and to your reduction of malpractice liability. Effective written communication in Nurses Notes is therapeutic for both patients and the nurses who author them.

We have previously discussed the potential advantages and disadvantages of computerized Nurses Notes. Now let's look at a new development that is even more immediate, less expensive to implement, and potentially more valuable to all health care members. This new form of written communication is called "Integrated Progress Notes," and they are important for several reasons.

1. Integrated Progress Notes are a single document that records physicians', nurses', dietitians', and therapists' (respiratory, physical, and occupational) information about a patient. It is a daily record of these multiple health care providers' interactions, assessments, interventions, treatments, and diagnoses on each patient.

2. Readers no longer need to turn to three or four different places in a chart to find various information about a patient's hospitalization.

3. Changes in the patient's care or condition are clearly obvious in such a record to all who use the document.

4. Information can be easily exchanged between a wide array of readers with a minimum of effort.

5. The risk of error is lowered since all readers have direct access to the same information.

The Oklahoma State Medical Association (1991) recently informed its members,

> Hospitals are being encouraged to consider going to integrated charting by the Loss Prevention Committee of the PLICO [Physicians Liability Insurance Company] Board of Directors. Such notes, where everyone with direct patient contact writes progress notes on the same sheet, are in use in many hospitals and have improved intra-staff communications dramatically, while lowering the number of order errors. (p. 1)

Indeed, the obvious advantages for physicians, nurses, and other members of the health care team would seem to outweigh any disadvantages. In fact, it is hard to imagine any disadvantages, other than the aforementioned problems with penmanship. However, if health care is truly a team effort, then written communication by and between members of the team should be consistent and contiguous in order to ensure optimal communication among health care professionals.

7

Discussion

PERSONALIZE YOUR COMMUNICATION

As we conclude our discussion, let us make a plea for you to never forget that patients are people, not diseases or injuries. Try to avoid the too often used references: "the gallbladder in 203, the hernia in 189, or the terminally ill woman in ICU." This type of depersonalized language serves to reinforce dehumanizing communication and behaviors. After all, if you're talking to a hernia, not a person, you don't need to really worry about transactional communication. Or if you're describing your interaction with the gall bladder in 203, not Ms. Talbot, then why worry about communicating her feelings and statements. (If you don't recall ever hearing such conversations, then just sit around medical personnel for a few minutes and listen to them talk about patients, then take a few minutes to listen to yourself talk about them.)

Try to always introduce yourself to your patients. Even in the E.R., patients are in vulnerable positions, and you are their representative. You wouldn't trust your child to a stranger, yet many health care workers expect patients to answer highly personal questions and undress and allow themselves to be touched, probed, and hurt by medical personnel who are often no more to patients than strangers. Do your best to give patients a name to go along with your face and treat them with respect by always referring to them by their surname, unless they give you permission to call them by their first name. And don't assume a woman is married just because she's over 20 or even because she's wearing a ring on the ring finger of her left hand. Be courteous and respectful and refer to men as Mr. and women as Ms. Patients will respect you for it, and you'll find them remembering your name and treating you with the same courtesy you extend to them. (Recall the principle of reciprocity we've discussed throughout this text.)

IMPORTANCE OF COMMUNICATION COMPETENCE

We have tried to stress the value of communication competence to every aspect of your work as a professional nurse. You need to be a competent communicator in order to interview and assess patients, to persuade them to trust you and cooperate with you in their care, and to get them to comply with your requests and their treatment plan.

Communication competence is also vital to the interactions that occur between countless members of the health care team. For example, nurse-doctor communication is critical to the assessment, care, and treatment of patients. In addition, the role of communication competence in nurse-nurse interactions cannot be underestimated. Without effective communication between professional nurses, there could be no continuity of care, and patients and their families would suffer greatly. Similarly, nurse-patient's family communication is critical to the exchange of information about a patient, to defraying unnecessary anxiety, and to the establishment of trust and credibility. Nursing professionals work closely with numerous members of the ancillary health care team: lab techs, X-ray techs, respiratory techs, physical therapists, and dietitians, to name a few. Without the cooperation of all members of the health care team, patients' suffering cannot be reduced and patient care cannot be readily advanced. As we've mentioned, nurse-supervisor or administrator communication competence is vital to the educational and professional goals of all who are involved. It is your responsibility to communicate effectively with your supervisors and administrators, and it is their responsibility to cooperate with you in assuring that patients are obtaining the best health care possible. Finally, communication competence helps to reduce your risks of malpractice litigation. Patients are less likely to accuse nurses who are respectful, supportive, compassionate, empathic, and caring. Your communication competence allows you to demonstrate all of these qualities to patients and, in so doing, you also display your professional competency and further your credibility.

THE FUTURE OF HEALTH CARE COMMUNICATION

We have all seen or heard about science-fiction movies with computers that store patient's medical records, use lasers to examine a patient, and then treat them on the spot. While there is no doubt that computers and technology will change the face of medicine greatly during the next 20 years, there is also one truth that can be just as assuredly attested to—health care will always need human beings to assess the complexities of individual patients. In other words, a computer may be able to pinpoint a tumor or localize a drop of blood inside an injured patient's brain, but the computer can't use transactional communication to interact with patients about their human responses to illnesses and/or injuries. Nor can a computer assist patients with the anxieties and concerns that illness and injury bring. Finally, a computer cannot tell when a patient's psychosocial illness is mimicking a biological one.

It is hard to imagine a world of health care without human communicators, and if you intend to stay in this field for another 10, 20, or even 40 years, you will no doubt see changes that we today cannot even fathom. You will probably also witness one great commonality between the health care of today and health care in the year 2031—there will still be nurses and patients who need to communicate with someone who is willing to listen, educate, explain, treat, and support. The role of transactional communication in health care of the future can only be expected to grow, not shrink, and your ability to effectively use transactional communication in your interactions will assure you a place in the nursing profession of today and tomorrow.

Health care in the year 2000 and beyond will almost assuredly require more accountability on your part. As health consumers see the costs of medical care soaring, they are going to demand more and more assurances that their medical dollars are being spent wisely. Your role in all this will blossom as you demonstrate, both verbally and in writing, how patients benefit from tests, treatment, and procedures. You won't necessarily have to describe the value of the test or treatment; rather, you will be expected to document how the patient's condition (the human response) has changed since receiving the treatment and thereby demonstrate its importance and economic worth.

Finally, communication competence is going to be critical in the years ahead because we are an aging nation, and as so many of us prepare for retirement and old age, we are going to be needing more and more nursing care away from the hospital. Such care will almost assuredly be delegated to nursing professionals at varying levels of health care delivery. From the hospital to the nursing home to the retirement village to patients' homes and beyond, we are going to need more and more highly trained, effective communicators to supervise the delivery of health care to the millions of Americans who will, within the next 20 years, be over 65.

Your ability to use effective verbal, nonverbal, and written communication can help you as you progress through all levels of professional nursing from the classroom to the bedside to the boardroom—remember to listen, observe, and exchange information, and you will have little difficulty demonstrating your competency and establishing your credibility as a nursing professional.

References

Afflerbach, D. (1986, January). A flow sheet that saves time and trouble. *RN*, 42-44.

Allport, G. W. (1968). Is the concept of self necessary? In C. Gordon & K. Gergen (Eds.), *The self in social interaction, Vol. I: Classic and contemporary perspectives* (pp. 25-32). New York: John Wiley.

American Nurses' Association. (1980). *Nursing: A social policy statement*. Kansas City, MO: Author.

Aristotle. (1960). *The rhetoric of Aristotle* (L. Cooper, Trans.). Englewood Cliffs, NJ: Prentice-Hall.

Bell, R. A., & Daly, J. A. (1984). The affinity-seeking function of communication. *Communication Monographs, 51*, 91-115.

Berger, C. R. (1985). Social power and interpersonal communication. In M. L. Knapp & G. R. Miller (Eds.), *Handbook of interpersonal communication* (pp. 439-499). Beverly Hills, CA: Sage.

Berlo, D. K. (1960). *The process of communication*. New York: Holt, Rinehart & Winston.

Bochner, A. P., & Kelley, C. W. (1974). Interpersonal competence: Rationale, philosophy and implementation of a conceptual framework. *Speech Teacher, 23*, 270-301.

Brown, P., & Levinson, S. C. (1987). *Politeness: Some universals in language usage*. Cambridge, UK: Cambridge University Press.

Burke, K. (1969a). *A grammar of motives*. Berkeley: University of California Press.

Burke, K. (1969b). *A rhetoric of motives*. Berkeley: University of California Press.

Burleson, B. (1984). Age, social-cognitive development, and the use of comforting. *Communication Monographs, 51*, 140-153.

Cicero. (1985). *De Oratore* (E. W. Sutton, Trans.). Cambridge, MA: Harvard University Press.

Connaway, N. (1985). Documenting patient care in the home: Legal issues for home health nurses. *Home Health Nurse, 3*(5), 600-601.

Cuzzell, J. Z. (1986). Tell it like it is: A realistic approach to wound documentation. *American Journal of Nursing, 86*(5), 600-601.

Dobberstein, K. (1986). Attacking fuzzy documentation. *American Journal of Nursing, 86*(5), 599.

Ekman, P., & Friesen, W. V. (1969). Nonverbal leakage and cues to deception. *Psychiatry, 32*, 88-106.

Feutz, S. A. (1987). Legal insights: Preventive legal maintenance. *JONA, 17*(1), 8-10.

French, J. R., & Raven, B. (1959). The bases for social power. In D. Cartwright (Ed.), *Studies in social power* (pp. 150-167). Ann Arbor, MI: Institute for Social Research.

Gondringer, N. S. (1986). Medical malpractice: The need for documentation/ communication. *Journal of the American Association of Nurse Anesthetists, 54*(6), 490-495.

Grove, T. G. (1991). *Dyadic interaction: Choice and change in conversations and relationships.* Dubuque, IA: William C. Brown.

Harkins, B. (1986, December). Keep your eye on the patient's problems. *RN*, 30-32.

Hopper, R. (1984). *Between you and me: The professional's guide to interpersonal communication.* Glenview, IL: Scott, Foresman.

Iyer, P. W. (1991a, June). Thirteen charting rules: To keep you legally safe. *Nursing, 91*, 40-44.

Iyer, P. W. (1991b, July). Six more charting rules: To keep you legally safe. *Nursing, 91*, 34-39.

Jacob, S. R. (1985). The impact of documentation in home health care. *Home Healthcare Nurse, 3*(5), 16-20.

Joint Commission on Accreditation of Healthcare Organizations (1991). *Accreditation manual for hospitals.* Chicago: Author.

Jones, E. F., & Nisbett, R. E. (1971). The actor and the observer: Divergent perceptions of the causes of behavior. In E. F. Jones (Ed.), *Attribution: Perceiving the causes of behavior* (pp. 79-94). Morristown, NJ: General Learning.

Jones, E. F., & Pittman, T. S. (1980). Toward a general theory of strategic self-presentation. In S. Trenholm & A. Jensen, *Interpersonal Communication* (pp. 218-220). Belmont, CA: Wadsworth.

Killian, W. H. (1991). Keep medical records accurate, timely. *The American Nurse, 23*(3), 22-23.

King, I. M. (1981). *Toward a theory for nursing.* New York: J. B. Lippincott.

Knapp, M. L., Cody, M. J., & Reardon, K. K. (1987). Nonverbal signals. In C. R. Berger & S. H. Caffee (Eds.), *Handbook of communication science* (pp. 385-418). Beverly Hills, CA: Sage.

Knapp, M. L., & Comadena, M. (1979). Telling it like it isn't. *Human Communication Research, 5*, 270-285.

Kreps, G. L., & Query, J. L. (1990). Health communication and interpersonal competence. In G. M. Phillips & J. T. Woods (Eds.), *Speech communication: Essays to commemorate the 75th anniversary of the Speech Communication Association* (pp. 292-323). Carbondale: Southern Illinois University Press.

Kübler-Ross, E. (1969). *On death and dying.* New York: Macmillan.

Manion, J. (1986, March/April). Developing a documentation system that works. *Journal of Obstetrics, Gynecology & Neonatal Nursing*, pp. 103-108.

Marwell, G., & Schmitt, D. R. (1967). Dimensions of compliance-gaining behavior: An empirical analysis. *Sociometry, 30*, 350-364.

Mathis, J. C., & Stevenson, D. (1980). Audience analysis: The problem and the solution. In K. J. Harty (Ed.), *Strategies for business and technical writing.* New York: Harcourt Brace Jovanovich.

McCroskey, J. J. (1977). Oral communication apprehension: A summary of recent theory and research. *Human Communication Research, 4*, 78-96.

McCroskey, J. J., Richmond, V. P., & Stewart, R. A. (1986). *One on one: The foundations of interpersonal communication.* Englewood Cliffs, NJ: Prentice-Hall.

Mills, G. H., & Walter, J. A. (1978). *Technical writing* (4th ed.). New York: Holt, Rinehart & Winston.

Morse, B., & Piland, R. (1981). An assessment of communication needed by intermediate-level health care providers: A study of nurse-patient, nurse-doctor, and nurse-nurse communication relationships. *Journal of Applied Communication Research, 9*, 30-41.

Oklahoma State Medical Association. (1991). *PLICO news.* Oklahoma City: Author.

Orlando, I. J. (1961). *The dynamic nurse-patient relationship: Function process and principles.* New York: G. P. Putnam.

Parsek. J. D. (1991) Did JCAHO abolish care plans? Yes! *The American Nurse, 23*(8), 2.

Peplau, H. E. (1952). *Interpersonal relations in nursing.* New York: G. P. Putnam.

Philpott, M. (1986, August). 20 rules for good charting. *Nursing, 86*, 63.

Prelli, L. J. (1989). *A rhetoric of science: Inventing scientific discourse.* Columbia: University of South Carolina Press.

Ragan, S. L., & Pagano, M. P. (1987). Communicating with female patients: Affective interaction during contraceptive counseling and the gynecologic exam. *Women's Studies in Communication, 10*, 47-56.

Reardon, K. K. (1981). *Persuasion: Theory and context.* Beverly Hills: Sage.

Reardon, K. K. (1984, March). Emotion and reason in persuasion. Paper presented at the meeting of the Central States Speech Association, Chicago, IL.

Reardon, K. K. (1987). *Interpersonal communication: Where minds meet.* Belmont, CA: Wadsworth.

Reardon, K. K., & Boyd, B. R. (1985). *Emotion and compliance in two types of relationships.* Unpublished manuscript, University of Connecticut, Annenburg School of Communication, Hartford, CT.

Reardon, K. K., & Boyd, B. R. (1986, May). Emotion and cognitive complexity in compliance-gaining. Paper presented at the meeting of the International Communication Association, Chicago, IL.

Reardon, K. K., & Buck, R. (1984, May). Emotion, reason and communication in coping with breast cancer. Paper presented at the meeting of the International Communication Association, San Francisco, CA.

Rhodes, A. M. (1986). Principles of documentation. *MCN, 11*, 381.

Rutkowski, B. (1985, October). How D.R.G.s are changing your charting. *Nursing85*, pp. 49-51.

Satir, V. (1967). *Conjoint family therapy.* Palo Alto, CA: Science and Behavior Books.

Scholes, R., & Comley, N. R. (1981). *The practice of writing.* New York: St. Martin's.

Sieburg, E., & Larson, C. (1971, May). Dimensions of interpersonal response. Paper presented at the meeting of the International Communication Association, Phoenix, AZ.

Sluzki, C. E., Beavin, J., Tarnopolsky, A., & Veron, E. (1967). Transactional disqualification. *Archives of General Psychiatry, 16*, 494-504.

Sullivan, C., & Reardon, K. K. (1985). Social support and health locus of control: Discriminators or breast cancer coping style preference. In M. McLaughlin (Ed.), *Communication Yearbook 9* (pp. 707-722). Beverly Hills, CA: Sage.

Thornton, L. A. (1986, April). We teach nurses to chart defensively. *RN*, pp. 57-60.

Tracy, K., Craig, R. T., Smith, M., & Spisak, F. (1984). The discourse of requests: Assessment of a compliance-gaining approach. *Human Communication Research, 10*, 513-538.

Trenholm, S., & Jensen, A. (1988). *Interpersonal communication*. Belmont, CA: Wadsworth.

Troyka, L. Q. (1987). *Handbook for writers*. Englewood Cliffs, NJ: Prentice-Hall.

Watzlawick, P., Bavelas, J. B., & Jackson, D. D. (1967). *Pragmatics of human communication: A study of interactional patterns, pathologies, & paradoxes*. New York: Norton.

Weeks, L. C., & Darrah, P. (1985). The documentation dilemma: A practical solution. *Journal of Nursing Administration, 15*(11), 22-27.

Wiemann, J. M. (1977). Explication and test of a model of communicative competence. *Human Communication Research, 3,* 195-213.

Wilmington, S. C. (1986). Oral communication instruction for a career in nursing. *Journal of Nursing Education, 25,* 195-213.

Wilmot, W. (1987). *Dyadic communication* (3rd ed.). New York: Random House.

Bibliography

Bergerson, S. (1988). More about charting with a jury in mind. *Nursing 88, 18*(4), 50-56.

Carkhuff, R. (1967). Toward a comprehensive model of facilitative interpersonal processes. *Journal of Counseling Psychology, 14,* 67-72.

Cassata, D. (1980). Health communication theory and research: A definitional overview. *Communication Yearbook 4,* 583-589.

Dance, F.E.X. (1982). *Human communication theory.* New York: Harper & Row.

DiSalvo, V. S., Larsen, J. K., & Backus, D. K. (1986). The health care communicator: An identification of skills and problems. *Communication Education, 35,* 231-242.

Feutz, S. (1989). *Nursing and the law.* Eau Claire, WI: Professional Education System.

Feutz, S. A. (1986). Nurses in the legal world. *JONA, 16*(10), 12-14.

Gibb, J. (1961). Defensive communication. *Journal of Communication, 3,* 141-148.

Given, B., & Simmons, S. (1977). The interdisciplinary health care team. *Nursing Forum, 16,* 164-184.

Gottlieb, B. (1981). *Social networks and social support.* Beverly Hills, CA: Sage.

Guido, G. (1988). *Legal issues in nursing.* Norwalk, CT: Appleton & Lange.

Korsch, B. M., Gozzi, E. K., & Francis, V. (1968). Gaps in doctor-patient communication: Doctor-patient interaction and patient satisfaction. *Pediatrics, 42,* 855-871.

Kreps, G. L. (1988). Relational communication in health care. *Southern Speech Communication Journal, 53,* 344-359.

Kreps, G. L., & Thornton, B. C. (1984). *Health communication.* New York: Longman.

Kübler-Ross, E. (1971). Dying with dignity. *The Canadian Nurse, 67(10),* 31-35.

Kübler-Ross, E. (1975). *Death: The final stage of growth.* Englewood Cliffs, NJ: Prentice-Hall.

Morse, B., & Piland, R. (1981). An assessment of communication competencies needed by intermediate-level health care providers: A study of nurse-patient, nurse-doctor, nurse-nurse communication relationships. *Journal of Applied Communication Research, 9,* 30-41.

Philpott, M. (1985). *Legal liability and the nursing process.* Toronto: W. B. Saunders.

Rossiter, C. (1975). Defining therapeutic communication. *Journal of Communication, 25,* 127-130.

Spitzberg, B. H., & Cupach, W. R. (1984). *Interpersonal communication competence.* Beverly Hills, CA: Sage.

Sudnow, D. (1967). *Passing on: The social organization of dying. Englewood Cliffs, NJ: Prentice-Hall.*

Thompson, T. (1984). The invisible helping hand: The role of communication in health and social service professions. *Communication Quarterly, 32,* 148-163.

Weed, L. L. (1969). *Medical records, medical education, and patient care.* Cleveland, OH: Case Western Reserve University Press.

Wilmington, S. C. (1986). Oral communication instruction for a career in nursing. *Journal of Nursing Education, 25,* 291-294.

Index

About the Authors

Michael P. Pagano, Ph.D., P.A., is Professor and Chair of the Physician Assistant Program at the University of Health Sciences/ The Chicago Medical School. He received his doctoral degree in health communication from the University of Oklahoma. His teaching interests include written communication, health communication, public speak- ing, and rhetoric. His research investigates natural settings in various health care contexts, most recently in the area of OB-GYN residents' training. In addition to his research and teaching interests, he works as a Physician's Assistant in a rural hospital Emergency Department and as a clinician for Planned Parenthood of Eastern Oklahoma. He has published several journal articles and has authored another textbook, *Communicating Effectively in Medical Records*, which is being published by Sage as well.

Sandra L. Ragan, Ph.D., is Associate Professor in the Department of Communication and in the Women's Studies Program at the University of Oklahoma. She received her doctoral degree in interpersonal communication from the University of Texas. She teaches interpersonal communication, female/male communication, and language pragmatics. Her research investigates naturally occurring conversations in a number of contexts, most recently in women's health communication. She is a former editor of the journal *Women's Studies in Communication* and has been published in that journal and several others related to language and communication. She has also contributed chapters to several books, the most recent of which discusses communication and gynecologic health care. She is currently engaged in a research project that explores the health care concerns of elderly women.

Deborah Booton, Ph.D., R.N., R.N.C., F.N.P., is Assistant Professor of Nursing at the University of Oklahoma in Oklahoma City. She obtained her doctoral degree from Texas Women's University, her master's degree as a Family Nurse Practitioner from Vanderbilt University, and her bachelor's degree from Oklahoma Baptist University. She is the project-director for a newly funded Advanced Nurse Education Grant and is working to develop and implement a Family Nurse Practitioner program within the existing University of Oklahoma master's program. In addition to her faculty position, she maintains her clinical competence by routinely working as a Family Nurse Practitioner in a hospital Emergency Department. She has con- ducted multiple workshops on documentation and physical assessment for nurses. Her research focuses on health behaviors related to hyper-lipoproteinemia, dysmenorrhea, and obesity. She is a co-investigator on a federal research grant involving the assessment of cultural norms and health practices among Oklahoma's Mvskoke Creek Indians.